THE FERTILITY BOOK

21 Days of Optimal Nutrition to Jumpstart Your Path to Pregnancy

Dr. Tamara ZumMallen, DAOM, L.Ac.

The Fertility Book ©Copyright 2023 Dr. Tamara ZumMallen, DAOM, L.Ac.

All rights reserved. No part of this publication may be reproduced, distributed or transmitted in any form or by any means, including photocopying, recording, or other electronic or mechanical methods, without the prior written permission of the publisher, except in the case of brief quotations embodied in critical reviews and certain other noncommercial uses permitted by copyright law.

Although the author and publisher have made every effort to ensure that the information in this book was correct at press time, the author and publisher do not assume and hereby disclaim any liability to any party for any loss, damage, or disruption caused by errors or omissions, whether such errors or omissions result from negligence, accident, or any other cause.

Adherence to all applicable laws and regulations, including international, federal, state and local governing professional licensing, business practices, advertising, and all other aspects of doing business in the US, Canada or any other jurisdiction is the sole responsibility of the reader and consumer.

The information provided herein is for informational purposes only and is not a substitute for medical advice, medical diagnosis, or medical treatment. Neither the author nor the publisher assumes any responsibility or liability whatsoever on behalf of the consumer or reader of this material.

The resources in this book are provided for informational purposes only and should not be used to replace the specialized training and professional judgment of a health care or mental health care professional.

For more information, email tamara@thefertilitybook.com

ISBN: 979-8-9853530-0-6 (paperback)

ISBN: 979-8-9853530-1-3 (eBook)

Get Your Free Gift!

As an added bonus to *The Fertility Book*, I have included a link to get immediate access to *The Male Fertility Book: A Companion Guide to The Fertility Book*, written to encourage male partners to be involved in fertility preparation.

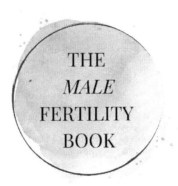

You can get a copy by visiting:
www.thefertilitybook.com

The Fertility Book is dedicated to all parents, especially mine.

Table of Contents

Foreword: Tamara's Story 9

Introduction. 11

Section One: The Forbiddens

Chapter One: Sugar 23

Chapter Two: Caffeine 27

Chapter Three: Alcohol 31

Chapter Four: Iced/Cold/Frozen Foods
                 And Beverages. 33

Section Two: Lifestyle

Chapter Five: Sleep 39

Chapter Six: Acupuncture 43

Chapter Seven: Exercise 49

Chapter Eight: Supplements. 51

Chapter Nine: Prenatal Vitamins 53

Chapter Ten: Coenzyme Q10 (Coq10) 59

Chapter Eleven: Vitamin D3 63

Section Three: The Plan

Chapter Twelve: The Plan. 69

Section Four: Recipes

Chapter Thirteen: Breakfasts 135

Chapter Fourteen: Lunches 147

Chapter Fifteen: Dinners 165

Chapter Sixteen: Sauces, Dressings, And
................Side Dishes 181
Notes 193
Acknowledgments 203

FOREWORD: TAMARA'S STORY

As a fertility acupuncturist, I have had the privilege of working with countless individuals and couples on their journey toward parenthood. The road to starting a family can be a difficult and emotional one, filled with hope, disappointment, and uncertainty.

Throughout my twenty-two years of practice, I have seen the profound impact that infertility can have on a person's life. It can cause feelings of isolation and sadness, depression and anxiety. It can strain relationships and test the strength of a couple's bond. It can make a person feel like they are less of a person, and invoke a sense of brokenness.

I have also seen the amazing resilience and determination of the individuals and couples I have worked with. I have seen the strength of their love and commitment, and the lengths they will go to to start a family. I have seen the hope that blossoms when people finally conceive, and the joy that fills a room when a baby is born. It is beautiful.

I have the honor of being a part of this journey, of supporting and guiding my patients through the ups and downs of fertility, infertility treatments, and ultimately bearing witness to dreams realized.

My role as a fertility acupuncturist is to provide the treatment modalities of Chinese medicine, acupuncture, and Chinese medicine-inspired nutrition to my patients with the goal of improving fertility and increasing the chances of conception. These modalities work by regulating the body's hormones and increasing blood flow to the reproductive organs. These modalities can also reduce stress and improve overall health, which can have a positive and profound impact on fertility.

Lifestyle counseling is an important aspect of my practice as well. I work with my patients to identify and address any lifestyle factors that may be impacting their fertility, such as exercise, sleep, and stress management. I also provide emotional support and guidance to help my patients navigate the rollercoaster of infertility treatment, from first preconception conversation through the postpartum period.

The Fertility Book is a guide to how fertility is approached in my acupuncture clinic. I hope that this book will serve as a valuable resource for anyone struggling with infertility. I am so excited to bring my clinic program to you. It is my sincere wish that the information and advice contained within these pages will help you on your journey to parenthood. Remember, you are not alone, and there is hope.

My most heartfelt wishes to you.
Dr. Tamara

INTRODUCTION

You are ready. You are hopeful. You are planning for the near future. But you got your period this morning.

Again.

This is when you phone my office. I will hear your disappointment, and my heart will break for you. But I have solutions—the research, recipes, and lifestyle wellness suggestions I have collected in these pages—that will help you as we try again. You catch your breath and smile, because you know I am here for you, whatever it takes!

Whether you have been struggling to conceive for a while or you have just started trying to get pregnant, I am so glad you chose this book to prepare for your miracle. Decades in the making, this book is based on the hundreds of conversations, thousands of meal suggestions, and countless acupuncture sessions that I have administered over the years with the intention of assisting in the creation of healthy, stress-free pregnancies.

When I began thinking about writing this book, I looked back at all the parents I have worked with and I asked myself if there was one common thread that connected them all. I would have to say it was the nourishment of body, mind, and spirit during the preconception period that truly made the difference. It is my hope that this book will help even more parents beyond my clinic walls make the most of the preconception period and gain a sense of control as they navigate this unchartered territory in their lives.

With over two decades of witnessing people becoming pregnant and carrying babies to term, I can honestly say the miracle is never lost on me. Every case is special. You are special. I want you to know that your story will have a beautiful ending.

There is a sacred space in between doing everything you need to do and allowing things to just happen: the middle ground, also known as being in the flow. In that in-between space, Mama, you will find peace. My number one piece of advice is to treat yourself as if you're already pregnant. Act as if it is true, and soon, the proposed suggestions in these pages will not feel so stringent. You will feel yourself in that in-between space, the flow.

So, let's prepare. Prepare to be pregnant. Prepare to hold your baby in your arms. Prepare to parent. Be kind and nurturing to yourself, right now. No matter what your story has been thus far, today is a day to begin anew. You may not be with me in my clinic, but I am willing to come to you in the form of this book. The things we talk about in the clinic, the way we prepare, it is all here, ready to help you, whatever you have been through so far.

Time and time again a person just like you has sat down in my office and said to me tearfully, "I've tried everything I can to get pregnant—what do I need to do?"

Well, start here!

In my acupuncture practice, we do not do bootcamps, cleanses, or detoxes, so my patients do not feel deprived or hungry. What we do is nurture and nourish, the Chinese medicine way. Whether you are planning on getting pregnant the good old-fashioned way or by using assisted reproductive techniques such as intrauterine insemination (IUI) or in vitro fertilization (IVF), Chinese medicine is the gentle persuasion you need. This is what we call "choosing the next best step," over and over, day after day, until you have formed the habits that will get you there. Every day, with every meal and every intention, we are choosing the next best step. It all adds up!

I wish I could fast forward for you for just a moment so I could show you just how okay it is all going to be. When you are weary and don't have faith, lean on mine. Experience has led me to have enough faith for both of us.

What I have for you in the pages of this book is a 21-day guide to a better-prepared you. I draw on the principles of Traditional Chinese Medicine (TCM), current research, and a whole lot of hope and encouragement.

This book offers a three-pronged approach: things to stop doing, things to start doing, and finally the complete 21-day guide. This plan will confidently take you from fertility novice to glowing, confident, preconception pro.

You will start each day of the 21 days by saying an affirmation and noting three things for which you are grateful. Throughout the day, you will practice self-care and consume delicious, nutrient-dense meals. At the end of the day, you are invited to write down your evening thoughts. I have found that affirmations, expressing gratitude, self-care, nutrition, and journaling are the perfect methods for success while trying to conceive. These methods help to create a positive and supportive mindset, optimize physical health, and manage stress levels – all of which can have a significant impact on fertility and the chances of conceiving. Affirmations can help to reframe any negative thoughts or beliefs around fertility and create a more positive outlook. Expressing gratitude can help to cultivate a sense of appreciation and contentment, which can improve overall wellbeing. Self-care practices, such as exercise and proper sleep, can help to reduce stress and support physical health. Proper nutrition can help to optimize fertility and support a healthy pregnancy. Journaling can be a helpful tool for processing emotions and managing stress, while also allowing for reflection and tracking of progress and goals. Together, these methods can provide a comprehensive approach to supporting fertility and the journey towards conception.

Why 21 days?

Experts say that it can take anywhere from 18 to 254 days to form a habit. Popular convention says 21 days, due to the work of surgeon Dr. Maxwell Maltz. In the 1950s, Dr. Maltz would perform amputations and plastic surgeries. When he asked patients how long it took for them to integrate and accept their new look, the average time was 21 days. He attributed this to the fact that it takes about 21 days for the brain to form a new neural pathway, or connection between neurons. He then published his findings in 1960, and the general public has accepted 21 days as a reasonable marker for change ever since.[1] In my clinical experience, at the three-week mark, people have grown comfortable with my suggested recommendations and changes. They feel great. These recommendations become progressively easier and start to feel sustainable. The change feels natural and most even get a jump on their pregnancy glow. Even the "forbidden three" (we will get to that in the next chapter) feel like a thing of the past after consistent effort over 21 days. So, if you can adopt these changes and stick with them for the 21 days covered in this book, you can confidently carry on *beyond* 21 days. I know you can.

Here are just a few case studies and fertility scenarios of people who have committed to the guidelines provided in this book and are now parents!

Jessica, 35 years old

Jessica was a professional dancer who had been trying to get pregnant for seven months. She and her husband decided that if they were not pregnant in the next three months, they would entertain the idea of intrauterine insemination (IUI). She was already doing most of the suggestions in *The Fertility Book*, but not diligent about supplements or refraining from sugar and caffeine. She came in just under her self-imposed deadline and became pregnant eleven weeks later. Her little boy is perfect!

Sarah, 40 years old

Sarah wanted to give herself the best chances to become pregnant during her one and only round of IVF. Sarah had one miscarriage and due to her age and history, wanted to go straight to IVF. She was referred to me by a friend who had had a similar case. She began the principles in *The Fertility Book* in conjunction with her prescribed infertility medications and made one perfect, genetically-tested embryo. Approximately five weeks later, she transferred this embryo. She had a wonderful pregnancy and gave birth to a perfect baby girl.

Theresa, 30 years old

Theresa knew she had time on her side, but wanted to prepare for pregnancy in the most effective way possible. In her words, her diet was "atrocious." She worked 50-60 hours a week. Sleep was an afterthought. The first thing that Theresa noticed after being mindful of her diet, and cutting out caffeine and alcohol, was a much-improved sleep pattern. *The Fertility Book* not only made her physically more healthy, it caused her to revamp her daily life. Eight weeks later she became pregnant and had a beautiful baby girl.

Angela, 36 years old

Angela had a history of recurrent pregnancy loss. After five miscarriages, she became weary of trying to conceive and fearful of how future pregnancies may progress. She and her husband decided to start the IVF process, but first wanted to give her body every possible chance at success. Admittedly, her diet and habits were not the best. She began *The Fertility Book* and became pregnant on her own, without IVF, seven weeks later. Her pregnancy progressed beautifully and she gave birth to a healthy baby boy.

I am so excited to take you on this 21-day journey. Without further adieu, let's jump into it.

SECTION ONE
The Forbiddens

I debated on whether or not to put the bad news first, but decided in the end that it would be best to rip the bandage off. Be forewarned: this section seems to be the most challenging part and the place where I get the most pushback in the clinic. When I mention abandoning sugar, caffeine, and alcohol, my patients all look disappointed. I understand. These things are all delicious, and some we equate with celebration. However, I guarantee you will notice you are having much more restful sleep after you eliminate sugar, caffeine, and alcohol. Just do your best and remember the big picture.

Taking steps towards eliminating harmful substances from your life can be a challenging but absolutely rewarding task. One important approach is to take it one day at a time, recognizing that change happens gradually. It is crucial not to overwhelm yourself by attempting to give up all three substances at once. Instead, focus on eliminating them individually, starting with one and then moving on to the next.

Allow yourself the time it takes to read this book, which typically spans a few days, and use this period as an opportunity to successfully eliminate all three substances one at a time. Remember, progress is a process, and by breaking it down into smaller, manageable steps, you can increase your chances of long-term success, even beyond the 21 days of this plan.

A fundamental aspect of this journey is finding healthy alternatives to replace the substances you are trying to eliminate. For example, when cravings strike, rather than reaching for a processed, sugary treat, consider opting for a piece of fruit. Not only will this satisfy your sweet tooth, but it will also provide essential vitamins, minerals, and fiber.

Similarly, if you usually enjoy a glass of wine to unwind, explore alternative ways to relax and find comfort. Instead of alcohol, try indulging in a hot herbal tea of your choice. Herbal teas have a calming effect and offer various health benefits.

For those accustomed to the energy kick of morning coffee, switching to a caffeine-free alternative like ginger or peppermint tea can provide a refreshing and flavorful start to your day.

Support from friends and family members is invaluable on this journey as well. Seek out an accountability partner who can join you in staying on track, motivating each other, and celebrating milestones together. Additionally, if you have a healthcare team, do not hesitate to involve them in your journey and ask for their support in holding you accountable. Many healthcare professionals are more than willing to review your habits, provide guidance, and even help you track your progress by reading your food journals.

As a healthcare professional myself, I frequently assist my patients in making these changes in their lives. I find great joy in offering support, reviewing their habits, and analyzing their food journals. Sharing your journey with someone who understands your unique challenges and is genuinely invested in your well-being can provide the extra boost you need to stay motivated.

Remember, embarking on this journey of change is a big decision, and while it may have its ups and downs, it will ultimately create a better-equipped and more prepared you.

CHAPTER ONE
SUGAR

Sugar is just about everyone's favorite vice. It makes food delicious and it is added in *everything*. Become a label-reader and you will see the sneaky way sugar has made its way into so many packaged goods. For the sake of this book, I took a stroll through the salad dressing aisle in the grocery store and found some form of sugar as one of the top ingredients in nine out of the first ten bottles I picked up off the shelf. Even options listed as low-calorie, fat-free, and generally healthier options contained sugar.

After that discouragement, I wandered over to the pasta sauce aisle. Same thing. Did I have better luck in the cracker aisle? Absolutely not.

You might not believe me, and that is because "sugar" is often hidden under other names on the label. Some other names for added sugar are: granulated sugar, table sugar, brown sugar, refined sugar, corn sugar, isoglucose, and high fructose corn syrup. Watch for these names too. My best piece of advice is to read every single label when considering a grocery store item.

What happens when you remove processed sugar from your diet? While much research is given to the adverse effect of excessive sugar consumption in pregnancy, the preconception period is just as important.[1] It is important to prepare for those very early days of pregnancy because some fetal organs have begun to form before some women are aware they are pregnant.

A study published in *Epidemiology* found that women who consumed more sugary drinks had a lower chance of getting pregnant. The study followed 2,674 women who were trying to conceive and found that those who drank one or more sugar-sweetened drinks per day, particularly sodas and energy drinks, had a lower chance of becoming pregnant in any given month compared to those who did not consume sugar-sweetened drinks.[2]

More research in the *The American Journal of Clinical Nutrition* found that high added sugar intake can lead to longer fecundability, or longer time to conception.[3]

Furthermore, sugar consumption has been linked to inflammation in the body. Inflammation is a natural response to injury or infection, but chronic inflammation can lead to a variety of health problems, including infertility. High sugar consumption has been linked to an increased risk of obesity, diabetes, hormonal imbalances, and other chronic health conditions. It is important for women to also consider the impact of sugar on their overall, long term health outside of pregnancy, and especially in the preconception period.

CHAPTER TWO
CAFFEINE

Caffeine is a widely used stimulant found in many beverages, including coffee, tea, soda, and even in chocolate. And we love it! It gives us a kick of energy in the morning and gets us over our afternoon slump. However, evidence suggests that high levels of caffeine intake can negatively impact a woman's ability to conceive. Women who are trying to conceive should avoid caffeine, as it has been linked to decreased fertility, increased risk of miscarriage, and low birth weight.[1,2]

Caffeine has also been linked to an increased risk of miscarriage. A study published in the *American Journal of Obstetrics and Gynecology* found that women who consumed more than 200 milligrams of caffeine per day had a higher risk of miscarriage compared to women who did not consume caffeine.[3] Findings in *International Journal of Obesity* note that high levels of caffeine intake during pregnancy can lead smaller birth weight, but obesity later in the child's life.[4]

During the preconception period and early stages of pregnancy, it is highly advisable to completely eliminate caffeine from your daily routine. While this may seem like a daunting task, I assure you that it is only temporary, and you will be able to indulge in all of your favorite caffeinated treats again in the future. To ensure a smooth transition, it is recommended to gradually reduce your caffeine intake, starting as soon as possible. It is important to note that abrupt cessation of caffeine consumption can lead to withdrawal symptoms, including headaches, particularly in susceptible individuals.

Understanding that headaches can be a potential side effect of withdrawing from caffeine, it is essential to be prepared for this temporary discomfort. Fortunately, in most cases, these headaches tend to subside within the first 48 hours of caffeine abstinence. During this period, prioritize hydration by drinking water throughout the day. Staying well-hydrated can help alleviate the intensity and duration of headaches.

By eliminating caffeine, you are safeguarding the well-being of your future unborn child, as well as setting the stage for a healthier pregnancy overall. Remember, this sacrifice is temporary, and once you have reached a later stage of pregnancy or the postpartum period, you can gradually reintroduce caffeine in moderation, under the guidance of your healthcare provider.

During this time, explore alternative beverage options that can provide comfort and satisfaction without caffeine. Opt for decaffeinated versions of your favorite hot beverages, such as herbal teas or caffeine-free coffee substitutes. Additionally, incorporating nourishing foods and snacks into your diet can help replenish the energy levels you might be missing from caffeine. I kept this in mind when I wrote the daily meal suggestions included in this 21-day plan.

CHAPTER THREE
ALCOHOL

The effects of alcohol on egg quality, follicular environment, and fertility have been the subject of many studies over the years, and the evidence suggests that alcohol can have a negative impact on all three.

Within the ovaries are follicles, the small sacs that contain immature eggs. In order for the eggs to mature and release during ovulation, a whole cascade of hormonal processes has to happen. Alcohol may hinder some of these processes. According to a systematic review and meta-analysis of 19 studies, alcohol consumption reduces a woman's chance of getting pregnant by 13 percent in any given cycle.[1] In addition to detrimental effects on follicular health, alcohol can lead to irregular ovulation, which can further reduce the likelihood of getting pregnant.

Consuming alcohol during pregnancy can lead to several health problems for both the mother and the baby. While this book addresses preconception care, I thought this was worth mentioning because some women are pregnant for weeks before they even realize it. You may fit into this category right now. One of the most severe consequences is fetal alcohol syndrome (FAS), which can cause developmental delays, intellectual disability, and facial abnormalities. According to the Centers for Disease Control and Prevention (CDC), there is no known safe amount of alcohol consumption during pregnancy, and even small amounts can cause harm to the developing fetus. Additionally, alcohol consumption during pregnancy can increase the risk of miscarriage, premature birth, and stillbirth.[2]

It is important to note that alcohol can have long-term effects on a child's development as well. A study published in the *Journal of Pediatrics* found that children whose mothers consumed alcohol during pregnancy were more likely to have behavioral problems, cognitive deficits, and lower academic achievement than children whose mothers did not drink any alcohol during pregnancy.[3]

In summary, women should avoid alcohol when trying to get pregnant to improve their chances of conceiving, reduce the risk of complications during pregnancy, and protect the long-term health of their child. It is crucial to note that these effects are not limited to heavy drinking and even moderate alcohol consumption can have significant negative consequences.[4]

You will raise a glass in celebration again at a later date. But for now, avoid all alcohol.

CHAPTER FOUR
ICED/COLD/FROZEN FOODS AND BEVERAGES

This chapter is unique to Chinese medicine, but I absolutely subscribe to this principle. Traditional Chinese Medicine (TCM) has a long history of promoting fertility and supporting healthy pregnancies with regard to food energetics and preparation. In TCM, it is believed that the body is in a constant state of balance, and that certain actions and behaviors can help maintain or disrupt one of the many things that are held in balance—for example, wet vs. dry, night vs. day, and cold vs. hot—and therefore affect our bodies as a whole. According to TCM principles, the human body is a complex system of energy channels that are responsible for the flow of energy and blood throughout the body. When these channels are blocked or disrupted by an imbalance, it can lead to a range of health issues, including infertility.

Our body temperature is what we will be focusing on here. Consuming cold foods is thought to have a cooling effect on the body and will disrupt the balance of yin and yang, the opposing yet complementary forces that are believed to make up the universe in Chinese philosophy.

Cold foods may be more difficult to digest, and some practitioners in Chinese medicine, myself included, believe that consuming cold foods can lead to subtle health issues. Cold foods can lead to stagnation of energy and blood flow. We never want to overheat or be too cold, especially when trying to conceive. Specifically, we think temperature change in the stomach may affect the womb's temperature, which can affect fertility.[1,2] One way to tell if an item is too cold for consumption is whether or not it is too cold to comfortably hold in your hand. Take iced tea, for example. If you need to switch the container back and forth from hand to hand because it is too cold to hold, then it is too cold for consumption. If an item gives you goose bumps or causes your teeth to chatter, it is too cold for consumption.

In addition to affecting energy flow, TCM teaches us that cold foods can also weaken the digestive system, which is responsible for processing and absorbing nutrients. When the digestive system is weakened, it can lead to nutrient deficiencies, which can further impact fertility. Take whatever measures you can take to prevent malabsorption, starting with avoiding cold foods.

It is worth noting that TCM is not opposed to all cold foods across the board. In fact, some cold foods are considered to be beneficial for certain health conditions. However, for the sake of fertility, it is generally recommended that women avoid cold foods altogether. You will notice the subtle warming effects of many of the recipes and diet suggestions I make later in this book.

In conclusion, TCM recommends avoiding cold foods when trying to conceive because they are believed to have a cooling effect on the body, which can disrupt the flow of energy and blood and cause cool conditions in the reproductive system. By opting for warm, cooked foods instead, women can support their fertility and increase their chances of conceiving, in TCM theory.

I hope you are convinced to halt the use of sugar, caffeine, alcohol, and iced/frozen foods and beverages. By refraining from these, you are taking significant steps toward improving your egg quality and overall health.

You might wonder about beneficial habits and practices to incorporate into your life while trying to conceive. In the next section, we will delve into that topic and provide insights and suggestions. The upcoming section addresses these important aspects of your journey to parenthood!

SECTION TWO
LIFESTYLE

This is not the part where I tell you to "just relax, and you will get pregnant." I promise.

You have already begun to create a more harmonious and fertility-friendly environment in your body with the suggestions made in Section one (eliminating sugar, caffeine, alcohol, and iced/cold/frozen foods and beverages). Let's add on—in this section, I want to address the ways in which it is possible to achieve a more relaxed state in your body, which, in turn, may help you to conceive.

When faced with stress, our bodies respond by releasing cortisol, a hormone that can wreak havoc on our overall well-being. Elevated levels of cortisol have been associated with a range of adverse health problems, such as elevated blood pressure, compromised immune system function, and unwanted weight gain. It is important to recognize that these negative consequences can interfere with the delicate balance of reproductive hormones.

To counteract these potential disruptions and increase the chances of successful conception, I often provide evidence-based suggestions to my patients. First and foremost, obtaining sufficient and restful sleep is paramount. Sleep plays a vital role in hormone regulation and overall physiological equilibrium. Additionally, incorporating practices like acupuncture, which has shown promise in reducing stress and enhancing fertility, can be beneficial.

Furthermore, engaging in regular physical exercise is not only advantageous for general health but can also alleviate stress levels and contribute to improved fertility.

Lastly, considering the judicious use of supplements may help address any nutritional deficiencies that could impact reproductive health.

By adopting these recommendations, individuals trying to conceive can take proactive steps to mitigate the detrimental effects of stress and optimize their chances of achieving a healthy pregnancy.

CHAPTER FIVE
SLEEP

Sleep is the foundation on which all of the other healthy habits are built. Sleep is the time to enter into rest and repair. Melatonin (relaxation hormone) is released. Cortisol (stress hormone) decreases. Gonadotropins (sex hormones) stabilize.

Getting enough sleep is essential for overall health and well-being, and it can also play a critical role in fertility. Sleep deprivation has been linked to several reproductive health problems, including difficulties in conception, low birth weight, and preterm labor.

A study published in the *Journal of Circadian Rhythms* found that women who slept less than six hours per night had decreased chances of getting pregnant compared to women who slept seven to eight hours per night. The study also revealed that women who slept more than nine hours per night had a decrease in their chances of conceiving. These findings suggests that the optimal amount of sleep for women trying to conceive is between seven and eight hours per night.[1]

More findings in the journal *Reproductive Biology and Endocrinology* looked at not only duration of sleep, but circadian rhythms and the importance of nocturnal sleeping. Their study corroborates numerous other studies confirming that babies of shift workers were more likely to be born prematurely and possibly with low birth weight.[2]

Poor sleep quality in both early and late pregnancy, may be associated with preterm birth.[3] While it is widely accepted that sleep becomes progressively more difficult and uncomfortable during pregnancy, it is important to establish adequate sleep habits in the preconception period, setting yourself up for more restful sleep in pregnancy, giving yourself the best chances at a full-term baby of adequate weight.

In addition to the amount of sleep, the quality of sleep is also important. Women who have trouble falling or staying asleep may experience hormonal imbalances that can affect fertility. Therefore, it is recommended to establish good sleep hygiene practices such as maintaining a regular sleep schedule, avoiding caffeine and alcohol, especially later in the day, and creating a comfortable sleeping environment.

One possible mechanism behind the link between sleep and fertility is the effect of sleep on sex hormones. Sleep deprivation can disrupt the balance of hormones that regulate ovulation, including luteinizing hormone (LH), follicle-stimulating hormone (FSH), and estrogen. These hormones play a critical role in the menstrual cycle, and any disruption in their balance can lead to irregular cycles and problems with ovulation.[4]

Another possible mechanism behind the link between sleep and fertility is the effect of sleep on stress levels. Quality sleep can decrease stress, while sleep deprivation can *increase* the levels of the stress hormones cortisol and adrenaline, which can interfere with ovulation and implantation. Chronic stress is defined as a prolonged state of psychological or physiological tension, and has been shown to disrupt the menstrual cycle and decrease fertility. Besides these physiological mechanisms, sleep also plays a significant role in a woman's overall sense of well-being, which in turn can impact her ability to conceive. Lack of sleep can weaken the immune system, making a woman more susceptible to infections and illnesses, which can also in turn affect fertility.

Improving sleep hygiene is essential in the preconception period. Some simple lifestyle changes around the sleep schedule will certainly help and contribute to the cumulative effect of all of your newfound, fertility-friendly habits. Here are a few of the habits you may want to incorporate:

- Stop consuming all food and beverages three hours before bed.
- Do something relaxing before bed, like read or make love.
- Pray, meditate, or set good intentions.
- Power down all electronic devices.
- Avoid watching television in bed.
- Invest in good bedding.

CHAPTER SIX
ACUPUNCTURE

Acupuncture is a 2000-year-old traditional Chinese medicine practice that involves the insertion of thin needles into specific points on the body to relieve pain and improve health. Acupuncture is my love, my passion, and my biggest contribution to fertility preparation. For the sake of this book I will keep it short and concise, but if you wish to take an even deeper dive into acupuncture for fertility, or if acupuncture care is unavailable in your area, I would recommend the book *The Infertility Cure* by Dr. Randine Lewis. Dr. Lewis has an excellent tutorial on the acupuncture points that are helpful when trying to conceive, and encourages self acupressure—perfect for women who cannot find an acupuncturist near them.

There are three specific reasons why you would want to incorporate acupuncture into your preconception plans:

1. Acupuncture increases blood flow to the uterus and ovaries. Acupuncture has been shown to increase

blood flow to the ovaries and uterus by dilating blood vessels and increasing the release of nitric oxide, a potent vasodilator. Vasodilation refers to the widening or relaxation of blood vessels, resulting in an increase in diameter. By improving blood flow, acupuncture may enhance the delivery of oxygen and nutrients to the reproductive organs, which may improve their function and overall health. A systematic review and meta-analysis of randomized controlled trials found that acupuncture was significantly effective in improving uterine blood flow and endometrial (uterine lining) thickness in women with infertility.[1] Another study showed that acupuncture increased blood flow to the ovaries and uterus in IVF patients with polycystic ovary syndrome (PCOS), a hormonal condition that is associated with reduced blood flow to the ovaries.[2]

2. Acupuncture, coupled with a proper diet, influences the hypothalamus-pituitary-ovarian (HPO) axis and how these organs and glands communicate with each other to produce hormones. The HPO axis is a complex hormonal system in the female reproductive system. It involves three main structures mentioned in its name: the hypothalamus, the pituitary gland, and the ovaries. The hypothalamus releases gonadotropin-releasing hormone (GnRH), which in turn stimulates the

pituitary gland to release follicle-stimulating hormone (FSH) and luteinizing hormone (LH). These hormones then stimulate the ovaries to produce estrogen and progesterone at specific times, which regulate the menstrual cycle, induce ovulation, and play vital roles in female fertility.

3. Lastly, acupuncture encourages relaxation and moves your body from sympathetic nervous response to a parasympathetic nervous response. Simply put, the body moves from flight or flight mode to rest and repair mode. Chronic stress can negatively affect reproductive health, especially in women; by promoting relaxation and reducing stress, this activation of the parasympathetic nervous system may help improve female fertility by creating a more supportive environment for reproductive function. It was reported in *Complementary Therapies in Clinical Practice* in 2022 that acupuncture was effective in reducing cortisol levels and reducing symptoms of anxiety and depression in patients with stress-related disorders.[3] Participants in this study reported reduced levels of stress, improved sleep quality, and increased feelings of well-being after receiving acupuncture treatments. Another way in which acupuncture encourages relaxation is with the release of endorphins, the feel-good hormones that help reduce pain. A study published in *Journal of Physics* investigated the effect

of acupuncture on endorphin release and mood in healthy volunteers. This study found that acupuncture increased endorphin levels in the blood of the participants.[4] How cool is that? One might expect to leave acupuncture sessions a little more relaxed, happy, and with less pain in the body.

When looking for a fertility acupuncturist, there are a few important factors to consider. First, make sure the acupuncturist is licensed and certified in your state or country. It is also important to look for an acupuncturist who has experience and training specifically in fertility treatment. Fertility acupuncturists readily provide this information on their websites. Additionally, consider the acupuncturist's approach and philosophy. Do they take a holistic approach, addressing lifestyle factors and emotional wellbeing in addition to physical symptoms? It is preferred that they do approach fertility patients holistically. Do they work closely with other healthcare providers, such as reproductive endocrinologists or OB/GYNs, to coordinate care?

Reading reviews and testimonials from other patients can also be helpful in gauging the acupuncturist's effectiveness and bedside manner. You may also ask your obstetrician/gynecologist or your reproductive endocrinologist for an acupuncture referral. They may have a list of preferred acupuncturists.

It is also important to consider practical factors such as location, availability, and cost. Finding an acupuncturist who is conveniently located and has appointment times that work with your schedule can make the process much smoother and less time-consuming. Finally, be sure to discuss any questions or concerns you have with the acupuncturist before starting treatment to ensure that you feel comfortable and confident in your choice. And once you have chosen an acupuncturist, tell your acupuncturist *everything* about your health and habits. For example, if you are experiencing sexual dysfunction, have a rash, or are indulging in recreational drug use, please say so. We won't judge! All details are helpful in creating your treatment plan. Remember, your acupuncturist wants you pregnant too!

CHAPTER SEVEN
EXERCISE

Exercise! Just a little. Just enough. When trying to conceive, it is not the time to start training for a marathon, but regular, moderate exercise has a positive effect on a woman's overall health, including her reproductive health, and may increase her chances of becoming pregnant. Let's explore the effect of exercise on women who are trying to conceive and the supporting scientific evidence.

Regular exercise can help improve a woman's chances of becoming pregnant. A study published in the *Journal of Basic Research in Medical Sciences* found that women who participated in moderate-intensity exercise had improved fertility compared to those who were inactive. The study suggested that moderate exercise can improve a woman's reproductive health by reducing stress and increasing blood flow to the reproductive organs, which can help regulate menstrual cycles and ovulation.[1]

Adding to the growing body of evidence of exercise and fertility, another study, published in the *Journal of*

Translational Medicine, found that amenorrheic women who exercised regularly resumed ovulation, and greatly reduced their incidences of infertility.[2]

While exercise can have a positive effect on a woman's fertility, it is important to approach exercise in moderation. Overexertion and extreme exercise can actually have a negative impact on a woman's reproductive health. According to a study published in the *Sports Medicine,* women who engaged in high-intensity exercise of more than 60 minutes per day, such as long-distance running, had a higher risk of irregular menstrual cycles, anovulation, and reduced fertility.[3] It is imperative for women to strike a balance between physical activity and rest, avoiding overexertion, and giving themselves sufficient recovery time.

In addition to the physical benefits of exercise, there are also psychological benefits that can impact a woman's fertility. Exercise has been shown to reduce stress and anxiety, which can—as we have discussed—have a positive effect on a woman's reproductive health. In this way, exercise offers the added benefits of overall well-being and psychological resilience.

If there is one form of moderate-intensity exercise I recommend above all else, it is walking. Walking is suitable for people of all fitness levels. Try walking four or five times a week, for thirty minutes per session. Ask your partner to join as a way of bonding and enjoying quality time together. You will both feel better taking these steps to help in the fertility journey. Pun intended.

CHAPTER EIGHT
SUPPLEMENTS

When it comes to maintaining optimal health, whole food nutrition is paramount for vitamin, mineral, and antioxidant purposes. Supplements, meanwhile, simply play a supporting role. We will discuss food and nutrition in the next section, but for now, this list of three supplements is both manageable and effective, and also will not break the bank. Getting pregnant should not send you on an expensive wild goose chase for products and ingredients that may or may not agree with you. It is feasible to take a more practical approach.

First and foremost, a prenatal vitamin should be first on your list. Packed with a comprehensive blend of essential vitamins and minerals specifically tailored to meet the unique needs of expectant mothers, prenatal vitamins provide an invaluable foundation for nurturing both the mother's health and the developing baby's well-being, starting in the preconception period.

Alongside prenatal vitamins, another indispensable supplement is Coenzyme Q10, also known as CoQ10. This remarkable antioxidant plays a pivotal role in neutralizing harmful free radicals, which can cause oxidative stress and potentially harm delicate cells. By incorporating CoQ10 into your supplement regimen, you empower your body with an additional defense against cellular damage, bolstering healthy eggs.

Last but certainly not least, vitamin D3 takes center stage in promoting follicular health, a vital aspect of the reproductive journey. With its numerous benefits, including enhancing follicle development and supporting hormonal production, vitamin D3 proves to be an indispensable ally for those seeking to optimize their fertility.

In the following chapters, we will explore each of these three supplements, shedding light on their unique properties, benefits, and recommended usage.

CHAPTER NINE
PRENATAL VITAMINS

The number one item on your supplement list is a prenatal vitamin. Taking prenatal vitamins before trying to conceive can help support a healthy pregnancy and reduce the risk of birth defects. Women who are planning to become pregnant should aim to start taking prenatal vitamins at least three months before conception. They should consult with their healthcare provider to determine if any additional supplements are necessary. If you have not done this already, start as soon as possible.

Ingredients vary, as do your individual needs. With so many to choose from—literally hundreds—this will be a conversation you need to have with your OB/GYN.

The American College of Obstetricians and Gynecologists (ACOG) offers the most comprehensive list of prenatal supplementation needs on their website: acog.org.[1,2] An effective prenatal vitamin will likely have many ingredients, but the foundation should be these four: folic acid, calcium, iron, and vitamin D3.

Folic Acid (600 mcg per day): The single most important ingredient in a prenatal vitamin is folic acid. Over 3000 studies confirm that folic acid is imperative in the prevention of neural tube defects. The neural tube is a structure that forms in the early stages of fetal development and eventually develops into the brain and spinal cord. The neural tube develops from a flat sheet of cells that folds in on itself to form a tube-like structure, with the top end expanding to form the brain and the bottom end becoming the spinal cord. The formation of the neural tube is a critical process that occurs during the first few weeks of pregnancy, typically between days eighteen and twenty-six after conception, before a woman even knows she is pregnant. If the neural tube fails to form properly or does not close completely, it can result in serious birth defects such as spina bifida or anencephaly. To prevent neural tube defects, it is recommended that women who are planning to become pregnant or who are in the early stages of pregnancy take folic acid supplements and/or consume foods that are rich in folic acid, such as leafy green vegetables, fortified cereals, and beans.

Calcium (1000 mg per day): Calcium builds strong bones and teeth in the child. Calcium is also responsible for aiding the prevention of preeclampsia (high blood pressure) in pregnancy. Calcium is an important nutrient for overall health, and it plays a particularly important role during pregnancy. Adequate calcium intake is necessary for a developing fetus to build strong bones and teeth, as well as for the proper development of the heart, nerves, and muscles. During pregnancy, the mother's body also goes through significant changes that can affect bone density. Calcium is needed to help maintain the mother's bone health during pregnancy, as well as to support the growth and development of the fetus. If a woman does not consume enough calcium during pregnancy, her body may take the calcium it needs for the baby from her bones, which can lead to decreased bone density and an increased risk of osteoporosis later in life. Therefore, it is important for women who are trying to get pregnant to consume enough calcium through their diet—and, if necessary, through supplementation—to support their own bone health *and* the healthy development of their growing baby. Some foods that are high in calcium are: leafy green vegetables, almonds, chickpeas, tofu, oranges, and figs.

Iron (27 mg per day): Iron is responsible for red blood cell development and oxygen delivery to the fetus. Iron is an essential mineral that plays a significant role in the body's ability to produce healthy red blood cells. When a woman is trying to get pregnant, taking iron supplements is recommended to help support her body's changing nutritional needs during pregnancy. During pregnancy, a woman's blood volume increases significantly, and her body needs to produce more red blood cells to support the growing fetus. Iron is a key component of hemoglobin, a protein found in red blood cells that is responsible for transporting oxygen throughout the body. Without enough iron, a woman may become anemic, which can cause fatigue, weakness, and other health complications that can be harmful to both the mother and the developing fetus. Taking an iron supplement before and during pregnancy can help ensure that a woman's body has enough iron to support the increased demand for red blood cells. Some iron-rich foods are: lentils, chickpeas, oats, spinach, beef, and eggs.

Vitamin D3 (600 IU per day): Vitamin D3 is an essential nutrient that plays a key role in reproductive health. In women, it helps to regulate the menstrual cycle, support ovarian function, and promote proper implantation of a fertilized egg. Additionally, adequate levels of vitamin D3 during pregnancy are important for fetal development, including proper bone growth in the baby and immune system function in the mother. Research has shown that low levels of vitamin D3 in women who are trying to conceive may increase the risk of infertility and pregnancy complications such as gestational diabetes and preeclampsia.

Some foods to consider to increase vitamin D levels are: fatty fish, egg yolks, mushrooms, and fortified orange juice.

CHAPTER TEN
COENZYME Q10 (COQ10)

The antioxidant Coenzyme Q10, also known as CoQ10, is a naturally occurring compound found in every cell of the human body, including the ovaries. It plays a vital role in the production of energy, as well as serving as an antioxidant that protects cells from oxidative damage. It is also responsible for keeping the ovaries' oocytes (eggs) fresh. An oocyte, the largest cell in the body, has about 100,000 mitochondria per cell. Mitochondria are orgnanelles within the cell that are responsible for producing energy within the cell, which is why mitochondria are sometimes referred to as the powerhouse of the cell. Mitochondria are also responsible for cell growth and cell death. As we age, and as oocytes are exposed to oxidative stress, the mitochondria become ineffective, rendering the egg "old" and less likely to fertilize. Regular CoQ10 may delay ovarian aging. It may even be possible to reverse age-related decline in egg quality.[1,2]

Studies have shown that a CoQ10 supplementation of between 200 and 600 mg per day can improve the quality of eggs, which may increase the chances of conception in women with polycystic ovarian syndrome as well as women with a history of poor ovarian reserve. A study published in the *Journal of Assisted Reproduction and Genetics* in 2020 found that CoQ10 supplementation improved egg quality in both groups of women who were undergoing in vitro fertilization (IVF) treatment.[3]

In addition to improving egg quality, CoQ10 supplementation may also help to increase the number of eggs that are available for fertilization. A study published in the *Reproductive Biology and Endocrinology* in 2018 found that CoQ10 supplementation increased the total number of viable eggs in women who were undergoing IVF treatment. Women who supplemented with CoQ10 for 60 days prior to the start of IVF treatment required lower doses of IVF medications. This may be particularly beneficial for women who have a low ovarian reserve, which can make it more difficult to conceive.[4]

It is worth noting that CoQ10 supplementation may also have benefits for men who are trying to conceive. Like women, men also produce less CoQ10 as they age, and this can have a negative impact on fertility. However, studies have shown that CoQ10 supplementation can improve sperm quality and motility (movement), which may increase the chances of conception.[5] For example, a study published in the *Clinical and Experimental Reproductive Medicine* in 2019 found that CoQ10 supplementation specifically improved sperm motility in men with infertility.

While more research is needed to fully understand the effects of CoQ10 supplementation on fertility, existing evidence suggests that it may be a safe and effective way to increase the chances of successful conception.

If you have purchased CoQ10 in the past, you may have noticed that it comes in two different forms: ubiquinol and ubiquinone. Choose the ubiquinol form. Ubiquinol is the more effective form of CoQ10 and is better absorbed by the body. While both ubiquinol and ubiquinone can provide excellent fertility benefits, ubiquinol is considered to be the more effective form of CoQ10 for fertility. This is because ubiquinol is the active, reduced form of CoQ10, while ubiquinone is the oxidized form.

Yes, this difference is really important. When we consume CoQ10, our body needs to convert it from ubiquinone to ubiquinol before it can be used. This conversion process becomes less efficient as we age, leading to lower levels of ubiquinol in our body. This is particularly relevant for women who are trying to conceive, as the quality of their eggs declines with age.

In addition to its fertility benefits, ubiquinol has also been shown to have a positive effect on overall health. It has been found to reduce inflammation, protect against oxidative stress, and improve cardiovascular health. This is also particularly important for women who are trying to conceive, as poor cardiovascular health has been linked to pregnancy complications such as preeclampsia and gestational diabetes.[6]

In conclusion, ubiquinol is the preferred form of CoQ10 for those trying to conceive due to its superior effectiveness. It has been shown to improve egg and sperm quality, increase the chances of conception, and reduce the risk of pregnancy complications. Supplementation with ubiquinol is a safe and effective way to support fertility and overall health. It is also important to choose a high-quality supplement from a reputable manufacturer to ensure that you are getting a safe and effective product. As with all supplementation, make your healthcare team aware of your plans to incorporate CoQ10 (ubiquinol) into your preconception plans.

CHAPTER ELEVEN
VITAMIN D3

We talked about vitamin D3 earlier in the prenatal vitamin section, but let's go a little deeper into vitamin D3 here, as it is recommended to take extra D3 during the preconception time in addition to what is already in our prenatal vitamin. Generally, dosage of vitamin D3 should be 1000 to 1500 IU (international units) per day, in addition to your prenatal vitamin.

The American College of Obstetricians and Gynecologists (ACOG) recommends that women who are pregnant or trying to conceive consume at least 600 IU of vitamin D daily, but do not specify an upper limit.[1] Optimal dose may vary depending on factors outside of diet such as skin color, geographic location, and sun exposure. A simple blood test given by your fertility doctor or OB/GYN will tell you if you are deficient.

There are vitamin D receptors in reproductive tissues, including ovaries, uterine lining, and placenta. Research also shows that vitamin D, over time, improves the follicular environment, resulting in better egg quality.[2] In women with polycystic ovarian syndrome and insulin resistance doing in vitro fertilization, vitamin D supplementation resulted in higher quality embryos and significantly higher pregnancy rates.[3]

The two different forms of vitamin D are vitamin D2 and vitamin D3. This fat-soluble vitamin plays a crucial role in maintaining bone health, immune function, improving fertility, and many other physiological processes in the body. But, vitamin D2 and D3 differ in their chemical structure and dietary sources. While both forms of vitamin D can be metabolized by the liver and kidneys to produce the biologically active form of vitamin D, known as calcitriol, there are some key differences between vitamin D2 and D3 that may impact their efficacy and health benefits.

Vitamin D2 (ergocalciferol) is primarily obtained from plants and fungi, and is produced by the UV irradiation of ergosterol found in certain types of mushrooms. It is also commonly found in fortified foods, such as cereal, milk, and orange juice.

Vitamin D3 (cholecalciferol), on the other hand, is primarily obtained from animal sources, such as fatty fish, egg yolks, and beef liver. Vitamin D3 is also obtained from lichen, a form of moss, which is of particular interest if you are looking for a plant-based option. Sun exposure is the most prevalent source of vitamin D3 for the body. However, it is important to balance the benefits of sun exposure with the risks of skin damage and skin cancer. Some experts recommend ten to fifteen minutes of sun exposure to the arms and legs (or face and hands) several times a week during peak sun hours.

Both vitamin D2 and vitamin D3 can be used by the body to raise blood levels of vitamin D, but vitamin D3 is considered to be the more potent and effective form. This is because vitamin D3 is more efficiently converted into the active form of vitamin D that the body uses to maintain calcium and phosphorus balance and support bone health.

Several studies confirm that vitamin D3 may be more effective at increasing circulating levels of vitamin D and improving health outcomes compared to vitamin D2. For example, a meta-analysis of 32 randomized controlled trials found that vitamin D3 was more effective than vitamin D2 at raising serum 25-hydroxyvitamin D levels, which is the most commonly used measurement of vitamin D status in the body.[4] Other studies that are indirectly related to fertility have also suggested that vitamin D3 may be more effective than vitamin D2 at improving bone health, reducing the risk of falls, and preventing certain types of cancer.

So, that is it for Section Two. Incorporating sleep, acupuncture (or acupressure), exercise, supplements, prenatal vitamins, CoEnzyme Q10 (CoQ10), and vitamin D3 can make significant improvements in your fertility journey. By implementing these elements, you are nurturing your body and providing it with the necessary tools to optimize your chances of conceiving. Remember to be patient and kind to yourself. With persistence and commitment, you will eventually get there. Trust the process.

Next up in Section Three is The Plan!

SECTION THREE

The Plan

CHAPTER TWELVE
THE PLAN

While there is no one-size-fits-all "fertility diet," I have developed the following recipes from a combination of my extensive knowledge of Chinese medicinal foods and foods with excellent nutritional profiles that will give you the most bang for your buck. In my hopeful heart, you will love every single recipe in Section Four.

The United States Department of Agriculture (USDA) has not published guidelines for women trying to conceive, but they have published guidelines for macronutrient (carbohydrates, protein, and fat) intake during pregnancy. A healthy preconception diet that emulates a pregnancy diet can help improve nutrient status and balance hormones, which may increase the likelihood of conceiving.[1] Additionally, a well-nourished mother can provide a better environment for the developing fetus long before she is pregnant, promoting healthy growth and reducing the risk of certain birth defects and complications during pregnancy.

According to USDA recommendations[2], pregnant women should consume a balanced diet that includes:

> Carbohydrates: Carbohydrates should provide 45 to 65 percent of total daily calories. Complex carbohydrates from fruits, vegetables, whole grains, and legumes are preferred over simple sugars and refined grains. Carbohydrates are an important macronutrient during pregnancy, as they provide energy for both the mother and developing fetus.

> Protein: Protein intake should be 10 to 35 percent of the total daily calories. Proteins are essential during pregnancy because they are necessary for fetal growth and development. Good sources of protein include lean meats, poultry, eggs, fish, tofu, beans, and nuts.

> Fat: Fat should provide 20 to 35 percent of total daily calories. Healthy fats from sources like nuts, seeds, avocado, and fatty fish are preferred over saturated and trans fats. Fats help with the development of the fetus's brain and nervous system.

It is important to recognize that these are general recommendations, and individual macronutrient needs can vary depending on factors such as pre-pregnancy weight, activity level, and any individual medical issues. It is always a good idea to consult with a healthcare provider or a registered dietitian for personalized recommendations.

In this plan, I will make daily meal suggestions, but you do not have to be rigid with the meal choices I have provided to see success. If you are the type of person who likes to plan and prepare your meals in advance for the week, most of these meals are ideal for you. You may prefer a few favorite recipes and choose them regularly. That is fine. Do not eat anything you are allergic to or that you simply do not like. If you see something here you find downright gross, do not eat it! Our palates are vastly different from one another, and that is okay. Meals should be enjoyed!

All breakfasts are interchangeable with other breakfasts, all lunches are interchangeable with other lunches, and all dinners are interchangeable with other dinners. Fresh fruits are interchangeable with other fresh fruits. Nuts and seeds are interchangeable with other nuts and seeds.

TCM leans away from vegetarianism and veganism as it considers these diets to be too cooling.[3] I understand that some people prefer these lifestyles. I have accommodated that and included some delicious vegetarian and vegan options. These meals will incorporate items with warming properties, such as ginger, cinnamon, onion, or garlic to offset the cold.

Noticeably absent from the recipes are dairy and gluten. One reason to avoid dairy products when trying to conceive is due to the presence of hormones in milk. Most cows are given hormones, such as bovine growth hormone, to increase milk production. These hormones can be passed on to humans who consume dairy products. Studies have shown that exposure to these hormones can disrupt the delicate balance of hormones in the human body, which may lead to fertility issues.[4] In one study, women who consumed low-fat dairy products had higher levels of anovulatory infertility compared to those who consumed less dairy.[5]

From the perspective of TCM, dairy products are known to be mucus-forming, which can lead to a buildup of phlegm in the body.[6] In Chinese medicine, this is seen as a sign of dampness, which can obstruct the flow of energy and blood to the reproductive organs.

Fortunately, there are wonderful non-dairy alternatives. At any supermarket, you will find: almond milk, coconut milk, hemp milk, oat milk, rice milk, and soy milk. All non-dairy milks will have a sugar-free option. Read those labels!

What is wrong with gluten? Some evidence suggests that gluten consumption may be associated with increased oxidative stress.[7] Oxidative stress occurs when there is an imbalance between the production of oxygen and the body's ability to detoxify, resulting in an excess of free radicals. This can lead to damage to cells and tissues, which can have a negative impact on fertility and pregnancy outcomes. By avoiding gluten, women may be able to reduce their exposure to compounds that promote oxidative stress and improve their chances of a healthy pregnancy.

I must mention again, it is important to note that these recommendations can vary depending on individual needs and health status. This is another reason to meet with a medical professional to assess your preconception needs, and to determine if you have clinical gluten sensitivity.

I have made this meal plan for you with *all* this information in mind. Each day meets the USDA suggested daily macronutrient intake—if not exactly, pretty darn close. Keep in mind, if you make any substitutions, your macronutrient numbers may skew a bit. My recommendation is getting an app that counts macronutrients and recording your meals there. There are *many* to choose from. Some of the popular ones I've come across among my patient population are: Lose It!, MyFitnessPal, My Plate, Macros, and Fooducate.

This section, Section Three, will go through the day-by-day 21-day plan; all recipes are in Section Four. I recommend that you open this book every morning for the next 21 days and say the suggested affirmation out loud or to yourself, and then note your gratitude, as the daily guide suggests. then take a deep breath and plan your day—complete with delicious and nutritious meals!

Why should I say a daily affirmation?

Affirmations are statements that are repeated frequently, usually to oneself. They are used to reinforce positive beliefs and attitudes, and to counteract negative thoughts and emotions. Affirmations can be used for reducing stress and anxiety, and enhancing overall well-being.

When we are feeling anxious or stressed, our thoughts can become negative and we may start to worry about things that have not even happened. Does this sound like you? If your mind starts to wander to a dark place, reign it in by saying your affirmation. It helps. By repeating positive affirmations, we can redirect our thoughts toward more positive and productive thinking patterns. This can help us feel more calm and in control, and reduce the impact of stress on our mental and emotional well-being.

When it comes to fertility, affirmations can be especially helpful. Trying to get pregnant can be a stressful and emotionally draining experience. People who are struggling with infertility may feel like they are constantly surrounded by negative thoughts and emotions. They may feel like their bodies are failing them, or like they are not good enough to be mothers. These negative thoughts and emotions can have a significant impact on a woman's fertility, as stress and anxiety can be disruptive to the hormonal balance needed for conception.

I have written affirmations for each day of the plan, but here are just a few more inspiring options:

"I am filled with hope and positivity today."

"My path to parenthood is unfolding perfectly."

"My body is strong, healthy and capable of conceiving a child."

"I release all doubts about my ability to conceive and carry a baby."

Repeating positive affirmations such as these throughout the day can help redirect our thoughts toward more positive and productive thinking patterns, taking the focus off what is around you and bringing the focus back to what is inside you. This can help you feel more calm and in control in the moment, as sometimes you are living your fertility moment to moment. Affirmations can also help you stay connected to your body and mind, helping to cultivate a positive attitude toward your fertility journey.

Why do I note my gratitude in the morning?

Gratitude is a powerful emotion that can have a positive impact on an individual's well-being and ability to achieve goals. Research has shown that cultivating gratitude can lead to improved mental health, increased resilience, and greater satisfaction with life.[8]

Researchers agree that practicing gratitude can change the brain's neural pathways and activate regions associated with positive thinking and wellbeing, ultimately leading to increased success and happiness during the day. A study involving infertile women found that regularly practicing gratitude and mindfulness can increase activity in the pre-frontal cortex, a region associated with decision-making and emotional processing.[9] This increased activity can lead to improved decision-making abilities and self-compassion, ultimately setting individuals up for success. This information shows us the need for addressing the psychosocial needs of infertile patients.

One of the ways in which gratitude can help with keeping positive is by promoting a more optimistic outlook on the little things in life, noticing the sacred in the seemingly-mundane tasks and rituals of the everyday experience. This can lead to greater feelings of happiness and well-being and provide an empowered start to the day.

In addition, gratitude can help individuals build stronger relationships with others. Expressing gratitude, even in written form, toward others can help to strengthen social connections and foster feelings of belonging and support. Mention your spouse, friends and family in your gratitude list. This, in turn, can contribute to a greater sense of positivity and overall well-being, and help to strengthen connection.

Gratitude can also help individuals overcome obstacles and setbacks that may arise in the preconception period. When individuals are grateful for the progress they have made, and every day there will be progress, they are more likely to persevere in the face of challenges and setbacks.

Here are a few examples of gratitude statements:

"I am grateful that my partner is on board with healthy meals to support our fertility journey."

"I am grateful for the list of friends I can call to express my concerns on particularly sad days."

"I am grateful for my daily walks because they get my blood pumping and my feel-good hormones flowing."

"I am grateful for that vast knowledge my medical team has and that they will be using that very valuable information to help me achieve a healthy pregnancy."

Give it a try. There are many things, big and small, to be grateful for. I have even made space in the 21-day plan to write your gratitude. Every morning, write down three things for which you are grateful. It is a quick and easy way to take care of your mental health, support your connections with others, and feel a bit more in control of the day ahead.

How will reflecting and writing down my thoughts at the end of the day help me?

One simple practice that can be helpful in managing the emotional toll of the fertility journey is taking time at the end of each day to reflect on the day's events and experiences with journaling.

Reflecting on the day can help individuals and couples on the fertility journey in several ways. It can help them focus on the positive aspects of their day, which can help to shift their mood and reduce feelings of stress and anxiety.[10] This can be especially helpful during times when the fertility journey feels overwhelming or frustrating. If the day's events weren't so great, get it out on paper. Tomorrow is a new day.

Reflecting on experiences can also help individuals and couples to cultivate a sense of gratitude and appreciation for the small steps you are taking in the right direction. This can be a powerful tool for building resilience and helping to manage the emotional ups and downs of the fertility journey, and the sometimes painfully long time it is taking.

Finally, taking time to reflect can help individuals and couples feel a sense of accomplishment and progress, especially on the days where there *is* significant progress, such as: getting a positive ovulation predictor test, getting the green light to start your IVF process, or planning an embryo transfer. Gosh, those days are special! By acknowledging these happy leaps forward, they can feel a sense of momentum and motivation to continue moving forward on their journey.

In conclusion, positively reflecting at the end of the day can be a helpful practice for individuals and couples on the fertility journey. By noting any and all aspects of their day, cultivating a sense of gratitude and appreciation, and acknowledging their progress and accomplishments, they can find strength, motivation, and resilience to continue moving forward. Additionally, taking time to reflect on positive experiences can help build intimacy and closeness between partners, strengthening your bond.

After your day is done, track any and all thoughts in the journal under the prompt "Tonight's Thoughts." I have reviewed the journals of patients in my clinic and some things they say worth noting are:

> cycle day
> symptoms
> intercourse
> what you are hopeful for
> notes to your future child
> what you are upset about
> exam and lab results of that day
> last night's sleep quality and quantity
> follicle count (if you're an IVF or IUI patient)
> positive interactions with healthcare professionals

I hope I have enticed you enough to commit to this plan. I am confident these 21 days will be easily integrated into your fertility life and you will want to implement these suggestions and keep going *beyond* day 21. Before you know it, your new habits will be a natural and effortless part of your daily routine. You might even get a head start on that beautiful pregnancy glow! Keep going.

So that is it! Day-by-day and sometimes, hour-by-hour, now we have a plan.

Are you excited? I am!

Day 1

"Faith is taking the first step even when you don't see the whole staircase." —Martin Luther King Jr.

Affirmation: I am committed to taking care of my body, mind, and spirit.

What are you grateful for this morning?

1.

2.

3.

Suggested Menu:

Breakfast: Green Veggie Frittata (page 135)
Midmorning Snack: 1 cup blueberries
Lunch: Chicken and rice bowl (page 147)
Afternoon Snack: 1/4 cup almonds
Dinner: Baked salmon with asparagus and cauliflower mash (page 165)

Day 1
Tonight's thoughts:

Day 2

"No matter how hard the world pushes against me, within me, there's something stronger, something better, pushing right back." —Albert Camus

Affirmation: My body is capable of conceiving and carrying a child.

What are you grateful for this morning?

1.

2.

3.

Suggested Menu:

Breakfast: Oatmeal with berries, ground flax seeds, and honey (page 137)
Midmorning Snack: 1 cup purple figs
Lunch: Bibimbap (page 149)
Afternoon snack: 1/4 cup walnuts
Dinner: Baked chicken with sweet and tart spinach (page 166)

Day 2

Tonight's thoughts:

Day 3

"Patience is the calm acceptance that things can happen in a different order than the one you had in mind." —David G. Allen

Affirmation: I am worthy of having a healthy and happy pregnancy.

What are you grateful for this morning?

1.

2.

3.

Suggested Menu:

Breakfast: Avocado toast with microgreens and black sesame seeds (page 138)
Midmorning snack: A piece of seasonal fruit
Lunch: Quinoa with chickpeas, spinach, red onions, and tomato (page 151)
Afternoon snack: 1/4 cup almonds
Dinner: Beef stew (page 167)

Day 3

Tonight's Thoughts:

Day 4

"She stood in the storm and when the wind did not blow her way, she adjusted her sails." —Elizabeth Edwards

Affirmation: I am filled with hope and positivity about my health and fertility journey.

What are you grateful for this morning?

1.

2.

3.

Suggested Menu:

Breakfast: Fried eggs with avocado and tomato (page 139)
Midmorning snack: 1 cup blueberries
Lunch: Lentil soup (page 153)
Afternoon snack: 1/4 cup walnuts
Dinner: Tofu stir fry with brown rice (page 169)

Day 4

Tonight's thoughts:

Day 5

"Hopeful thinking can get you out of your fear zone and into your appreciation zone." —Martha Beck

Affirmation: I release any stress or anxiety related to my fertility and health.

What are you grateful for this morning?

1.

2.

3.

Suggested Menu:

Breakfast: Muesli with almond milk, chia seeds, and goji berries (page 140)
Midmorning snack: 1 cup purple figs
Lunch: Green salad with chicken (page 155)
Afternoon snack: 1/4 cup almonds
Dinner: Quinoa with arugula, sweet potato, avocado, and eggs (page 171)

Day 5

Tonight's Thoughts:

Day 6

"The magic is inside you. There ain't no crystal ball." —Dolly Parton

Affirmation: I am open and receptive to the abundance of health and fertility in my life.

What are you grateful for this morning?

1.

2.

3.

Suggested Menu:

Breakfast: Foxtail millet porridge (page 141)
Midmorning snack: 1 piece of seasonal fruit
Lunch: Roasted veggies and tempeh over rice (page 157)
Afternoon snack: 1/4 cup walnuts
Dinner: Pan-seared steak salad (page 173)

Day 6

Tonight's Thoughts:

Day 7

"Try every avenue; try anything you can, 'cause you'll get there. You'll end up with a family, and it's so worth it. It is the most 'worth it' thing." —Jimmy Fallon

Affirmation: I am confident in my body's ability to create and sustain life.

What are you grateful for this morning?

1.

2.

3.

Suggested Menu:

Breakfast: Oatmeal bake (page 142)
Midmorning snack: 1 cup blueberries
Lunch: Grilled tofu bowl with tahini dressing (page 159)
Afternoon snack: 1/4 cup almonds
Dinner: Lamb stew with dates and sweet potatoes (page 175)

Day 7

Tonight's Thoughts:

WEEK ONE REFLECTION

You have completed one week. You should be proud of yourself! For most people, it is not easy to eliminate caffeine, sugar, and alcohol.

What was easiest for you?

What did you find most challenging?

Day 8

"There is such a special sweetness in being able to participate in creation." —Pamela S. Nadav

Affirmation: I like knowing that I am becoming more fertile.

What are you grateful for this morning?

1.

2.

3.

Suggested Menu:

Breakfast: Oatmeal with pumpkin, pecans, and ground flax seeds (page 144)
Midmorning snack: 1 cup purple figs
Lunch: Beet and chicken salad (page 161)
Afternoon snack: 1/4 cup walnuts
Dinner: Pan-seared steak with portobello mushrooms and zucchini (page 177)

Day 8

Tonight's Thoughts:

Day 9

"Be healthy and take care of yourself, but be happy with the beautiful things that make you, you." —Beyonce Knowles

Affirmation: I release any negative thoughts or beliefs about my fertility.

What are you grateful for this morning?

1.

2.

3.

Suggested Menu:

Breakfast: Almond butter toast with banana (page 146)
Midmorning snack: 1 piece of seasonal fruit
Lunch: Quinoa with arugula, sweet potatoes, and pomegranate (page 163)
Afternoon snack: 1/4 cup almonds
Dinner: Veggie stir fry with almonds (page 178)

Day 9

Tonight's Thoughts:

Day 10

"What we don't need in the midst of struggle is shame for being human." —Brené Brown

Affirmation: I am grateful for the wisdom of those who have gone before me on this journey.

What are you grateful for this morning?

1.

2.

3.

Suggested Menu:

Breakfast: Green veggie frittata (page 135)
Midmorning snack: 1 cup blueberries
Lunch: Chicken and rice bowl (page 147)
Afternoon snack: 1/4 cup walnuts
Dinner: Baked salmon with asparagus and cauliflower mash (page 165)

Day 10

Tonight's Thoughts:

Day 11

"The longer you hang in there, the greater the chance that something will happen in your favor." —Jack Canfield

Affirmation: I am worthy of experiencing the joys of parenthood.

What are you grateful for this morning?

1.

2.

3.

Suggested Menu:

Breakfast: Oatmeal with berries, ground flax seeds, and honey (page 137)
Midmorning snack: 1 cup purple figs
Lunch: Bibimbap (page 149)
Afternoon snack: 1/4 cup almonds
Dinner: Baked chicken with sweet and tart spinach (page 166)

Day 11

Tonight's Thoughts:

Day 12

"Always believe that something wonderful is about to happen."
—Dr. Sukhraj Dhillon

Affirmation: I am grateful for the abundance of resources available to me on my fertility journey.

What are you grateful for this morning?

1.

2.

3.

Suggested Menu:

Breakfast: Avocado toast with microgreens and black sesame seeds (page 138)
Midmorning snack: 1 piece of seasonal fruit
Lunch: Quinoa with chickpeas, spinach, red onions, and tomato (page 151)
Afternoon snack: 1/4 cup walnuts
Dinner: Beef stew (page 167)

Day 12

Tonight's Thoughts:

Day 13

"The moment you're ready to quit is usually the moment right before the miracle happens." —Unknown

Affirmation: I am confident in my ability to make healthy, informed decisions for my body.

What are you grateful for this morning?

1.

2.

3.

Suggested Menu:

Breakfast: Fried eggs with avocado and tomato (page 139)
Midmorning snack: 1 cup blueberries
Lunch: Lentil soup (page 153)
Afternoon snack: 1/4 cup almonds
Dinner: Tofu stir fry with brown rice (page 169)

Day 13

Tonight's Thoughts:

Day 14

"Don't give up before the future comes around that was meant for you, okay?" —Tara Wine-Queen

Affirmation: I am relaxed knowing that my journey is unique.

What are you grateful for this morning?

1.

2.

3.

Suggested Menu:

Breakfast: Muesli with almond milk, chia seeds, and goji berries (page 140)
Midmorning snack: 1 cup purple figs
Lunch: Green salad with chicken (page 155)
Afternoon snack: 1/4 cup walnuts
Dinner: Quinoa with arugula, sweet potato, avocado, and eggs (page 171)

Day 14

Tonight's Thoughts:

WEEK TWO REFLECTION

You are two-thirds of the way there. This is getting easier, right? If not, that is okay. You are doing your best and you should be proud. All of your efforts, even the little ones, will add up. Keep going! Your morning gratitude list rocks, doesn't it? It is okay if you list the same three sources of gratitude repeatedly. This simply reinforces the joy these bring you.

What was easiest for you?

What was hardest for you?

How has this changed from week one?

Day 15

"There is so much stubborn hope in the human heart."
—Albert Camus

Affirmation: I trust my body to create the biggest miracle of my life.

What are you grateful for this morning?

1.

2.

3.

Suggested Menu:

Breakfast: Foxtail millet porridge (page 141)
Midmorning snack: 1 piece of seasonal fruit
Lunch: Roasted veggies and tempeh over rice (page 157)
Afternoon snack: 1/4 cup almonds
Dinner: Pan-seared steak salad (page 173)

Day 15

Tonight's Thoughts:

Day 16

"Life is tough, my darling, but so are you."
—*Stephanie Bennett Henry*

Affirmation: I am grateful for the abundance of love and support that surrounds me.

What are you grateful for this morning?

1.

2.

3.

Suggested Menu:

Breakfast: Oatmeal bake (page 142)
Midmorning snack: 1 cup blueberries
Lunch: Grilled tofu bowl with tahini dressing (page 159)
Afternoon snack: 1/4 cup walnuts
Dinner: Lamb stew with dates and sweet potatoes (page 175)

Day 16

Tonight's Thoughts:

Day 17

"Just keep swimming." —Finding Nemo (2003)

Affirmation: I am worthy of experiencing all the joys that parenthood has to offer.

What are you grateful for this morning?

1.

2.

3.

Suggested Menu:

Breakfast: Oatmeal with pumpkin, pecans, and ground flax seeds (page 144)
Midmorning snack: 1 cup purple figs
Lunch: Beet and chicken salad (page 161)
Afternoon snack: 1/4 cup almonds
Dinner: Pan-seared steak with roasted portobello mushrooms and zucchini (page 177)

Day 17

Tonight's Thoughts:

Day 18

"Life loves to be taken by the lapel and told, 'I'm with you, kid. Let's go.'" —Maya Angelou

Affirmation: I am open to seeking support and guidance from professionals when needed.

What are you grateful for this morning?

1.

2.

3.

Suggested Menu:

Breakfast: Almond butter toast with banana (page 146)
Midmorning snack: 1 piece of seasonal fruit
Lunch: Quinoa with arugula, sweet potatoes, and pomegranate (page 163)
Afternoon snack: 1/4 cup walnuts
Dinner: Veggie stir fry with almonds (page 178)

Day 18

Tonight's Thoughts:

Day 19

"I inhale hope with every breath I take."
—Sharon Kay Penman

Affirmation: I am in awe at my body's ability to create life.

What are you grateful for this morning?

1.

2.

3.

Suggested Menu:

Breakfast: Green veggie frittata (page 135)
Midmorning snack: 1 cup blueberries
Lunch: Chicken and rice bowl (page 147)
Afternoon snack: 1/4 cup almonds
Dinner: Baked salmon with asparagus and cauliflower mash (page 165)

Day 19

Tonight's Thoughts:

Day 20

"Even miracles take a little time." —Cinderella (1950)

Affirmation: I am open to exploring all options and finding the right path on my unique fertility journey.

What are you grateful for this morning?

1.

2.

3.

Suggested Menu:

Breakfast: Avocado toast with microgreens and black sesame seeds (page 138)
Midmorning snack: 1 cup purple figs
Lunch: Bibimbap (page 149)
Afternoon snack: 1/4 cup walnuts
Dinner: Baked chicken with sweet and tart spinach (page 166)

Day 20

Tonight's Thoughts:

Day 21

"Babies bring angels."—Tamara ZumMallen

Affirmation: I know my turn to conceive is coming soon.

What are you grateful for this morning?

1.

2.

3.

Suggested Menu:

Breakfast: Fried eggs with avocado and tomato (page 139)
Midmorning snack: 1 piece of seasonal fruit
Lunch: Quinoa with chickpeas, spinach, red onions, and tomato (page 151)
Afternoon snack: 1/4 cup almonds
Dinner: Beef stew (page 167)

Day 21

Tonight's Thoughts:

WEEK THREE REVIEW AND FINAL THOUGHTS

You did it! You completed three weeks of habits, rituals, and nutrition that will help you turn a corner in your fertility journey. I am proud of you, but more importantly, you should be proud of yourself.

As you come to the final pages of this fertility book, it is my hope that the information and advice provided within these pages have been valuable to you on your journey to parenthood. I understand that trying to conceive can be an emotional and challenging experience, but I hope that the knowledge and insights shared in this book have provided you with the empowerment and confidence in yourself that you need to complete this journey.

The path you are on is shared by many. You are not alone and there are many resources available to you as you move forward. Whether it be seeking medical assistance, or alternative treatments, there is more than one path to parenthood. Stay open and find what path works for you.

I sincerely hope that this book has provided you with the springboard you were searching for to a more fertile you. I wholeheartedly encourage you to continue learning and seeking out experts, additional resources, and like-minded individuals as you navigate this journey. Remember, dear reader, that you are not alone in your pursuit. Community can provide solace, strength, and encouragement.

I wish you the very best. From the bottom of my heart, I do. I wish you profound joy in the discovery of two pink lines. I wish you camaraderie and support in your pregnancy journey. I wish you 3:00 a.m. feedings and the intoxicating scent of a newborn baby's crown. I wish you gummy smiles, coos, and cuddles. Most of all, I wish that your whole experience, from positive test to babe in your arms, is blissful.

Pat yourself on the back, document your pride here, keep going, and don't be shy to share your progress with me: https://www.facebook.com/thefertilitybook.

SECTION FOUR
Recipes

Recipes

Welcome to the recipe section of *The Fertility Book*. In this section, you will find a collection of recipes curated by me! I love to cook. To me, food is love. These recipes are carefully crafted to incorporate ingredients that are rich in the nutrients, vitamins, and minerals that are essential for reproductive health.

Bon Appétit!

Breakfasts:
Green veggie frittata - vegetarian (page 135)
Oatmeal with berries, ground flax seeds, and honey - vegetarian (page 137)
Avocado toast with microgreens and black sesame seeds - vegan (page 138)
Fried eggs with avocado and tomato - vegetarian (page 139)
Muesli with almond milk, chia seeds, and goji berries - vegan (page 140)
Foxtail millet porridge - vegan (page 141)
Oatmeal bake - vegetarian (page 142)
Oatmeal with pumpkin, pecans, and ground flax seeds - vegetarian (page 144)
Almond butter toast with banana - vegetarian (page 146)

Lunches:

Chicken and rice bowl (page 147)

Bibimbap (page 149)

Quinoa with chickpeas, spinach, red onions, and tomato - vegan (page 151)

Lentil soup - vegan (page 153)

Green salad with chicken (page 155)

Roasted veggies and tempeh over rice - vegan (page 157)

Grilled tofu bowl with tahini dressing - vegan (page 159)

Beet and chicken salad (page 161)

Quinoa with arugula, sweet potatoes, and pomegranate - vegan (page 163)

Dinners:

Baked salmon with asparagus and cauliflower mash (page 165)

Grilled chicken with sweet and tart spinach (page 166)

Beef stew (page 167)

Tofu stir fry with brown rice - vegan (page 169)

Quinoa with arugula, sweet potato, avocado, and eggs - vegetarian (page 171)

Pan-seared steak salad (page 173)

Lamb stew with dates and sweet potatoes (page 175)

Pan-seared steak with portobello mushrooms and zucchini (page 177)

Veggie stir fry with almonds - vegan (page 178)

Sauces and Dressings:

Tahini dressing (page 181)

Tangy orange dressing (page 182)

Simple vinaigrette dressing (page 183)

Parsley sauce (page 184)

Honey Dijon dressing (page 184)

Tamara's Marinade (page 185)

Side dishes:

Cauliflower mash (page 186)

Roasted portobello mushrooms and zucchini (page 187)

Roasted beets (page 188)

Roasted sweet potatoes (page 189)

Steamed asparagus (page 190)

Sweet and tart spinach (page 191)

CHAPTER THIRTEEN
BREAKFASTS

Green veggie frittata (Serves 4–6)

Ingredients:
- 8 large eggs
- 1 large handful of spinach
- 1 cup broccoli florets
- 10 asparagus stalks
- 1/4 yellow onion
- 2 Tbsp. avocado oil
- 2 cloves garlic, minced
- one pinch baking soda (optional)

Instructions:
1. Preheat your oven to 375°F.
2. In a medium bowl, whisk together the eggs, salt, and pepper until well combined. Add a pinch of baking soda (optional) for a fluffier frittata. Set aside.
3. In a large, oven-safe skillet (preferably non-stick), heat the avocado oil over medium heat.
4. Add the chopped onion and minced garlic. Sauté for 2–3 minutes until the onion is translucent and fragrant.

5. Add the spinach, broccoli, and asparagus to the skillet. Sauté for 5–7 minutes until they are tender and any excess water has evaporated.
6. Distribute veggies evenly in the pan, then pour in the egg mixture.
7. Cook on the stovetop for 2–3 minutes until the edges of the frittata start to set.
8. Transfer the skillet to the preheated oven. Bake for 10–15 minutes until the eggs are set.
9. Remove the skillet from the oven and let the frittata cool for a few minutes before slicing and serving.

Oatmeal with berries, ground flax seeds, and honey
(Serves 2)

Ingredients:
- 1 cup rolled oats
- 2 cups water
- pinch of salt
- 2 Tbsp. ground flaxseeds
- 1 tsp. cinnamon
- 1/2 cup blackberries
- 1/2 cup raspberries
- Honey (or vegan options: maple syrup or agave nectar)

Instructions:
1. In a medium-sized pot, combine the oats, water, and salt. Bring to a boil, then reduce the heat to low and simmer for 10–15 minutes, or until the oatmeal has thickened to your desired consistency.
2. Once the oatmeal is cooked, stir in the ground flaxseeds and cinnamon.
3. Divide the oatmeal into two bowls and top with berries.
4. Drizzle honey on top.

Adjust the sweetness to your liking by adding more or less honey, and you can also swap out the mixed berries for your favorite fruit.

Avocado toast with microgreens and black sesame seeds (Serves 1)

Ingredients:
- 1/2 ripe avocado
- 2 slices of gluten-free bread*
- A handful of microgreens
- 1/2 Tbsp. of black sesame seeds
- Salt and pepper to taste
- Lemon juice (optional)

Instructions:
1. Cut the avocado in half, remove the pit, and scoop out the flesh into a bowl.
2. Mash the avocado with a fork until it is smooth.
3. Add salt and pepper to taste, and a squeeze of lemon juice if desired.
4. Toast the slices of bread.
5. Spread the mashed avocado on top of the toast.
6. Sprinkle the microgreens and black sesame seeds on top of the avocado.
7. Serve and enjoy!

You can also add other ingredients to your avocado toast, such as sliced tomatoes, slices radishes, or a poached egg. Get creative and make it your own!

*Some favorite brands for gluten-free bread: Udi's, Canyon Bakehouse, Food For Life, Against The Grain.

Fried eggs with avocado and tomato (Serves 1)

Ingredients:
- 2 large eggs
- 1/2 ripe avocado
- 1/2 medium heirloom tomato
- 1 Tbsp. avocado oil
- Salt and pepper to taste

Instructions:
1. Slice the tomato and avocado into thin slices. Set aside.
2. Heat a non-stick frying pan over medium heat and add the avocado oil.
3. Crack eggs into a frying pan. Season the eggs with salt and pepper to taste and cook for 2–3 minutes until the whites are set and the yolks are cooked to your desired level of doneness.
4. While the eggs are cooking, arrange the avocado and tomato slices on a plate.
5. Once the eggs are cooked, use a spatula to carefully transfer them onto the plate with the tomato and avocado slices.
6. Serve immediately and enjoy!

You can also toast gluten-free bread to serve alongside the eggs if desired.

Muesli with almond milk, chia seeds, and goji berries (Serves 1)

Ingredients:
- 1 cup store bought muesli*
- 3/4 cup almond milk or other milk alternative
- 1/4 cup goji berries**
- 1 Tbsp. chia seeds

Instructions:
1. Put muesli in a bowl.
2. Pour almond milk over.
3. Sprinkle in goji berries and chia seeds and stir.
4. Serve immediately and enjoy!

*Some favorite store-bought muesli brands: Bob's Red Mill, Alpen, Seven Sundays, and Guud.

**Goji berries can be an acquired taste. If you find yourself liking the taste of the goji berries, but not the texture, try soaking them overnight in water for a softer texture. Substitute with blueberries if you really do not like goji berries.

Foxtail millet porridge (Serves 2)

Ingredients:
- 1 cup foxtail millet
- 4 cups water
- 1/2 tsp. salt
- 1/2 cup unsweetened almond milk (optional)
- Honey, agave nectar, or maple syrup, to taste
- Fresh fruits and nuts of your choice

Instructions:
1. Rinse the foxtail millet in a fine-mesh sieve or colander and drain well.
2. In a medium-sized pot, bring the water and salt to a boil. Add the foxtail millet, reduce the heat to low, and simmer for 20–25 minutes or until the millet is tender and the water is absorbed.
3. Stir in the almond milk (optional). Heat the porridge until hot.
4. Remove from the heat and stir in honey, agave nectar, or maple syrup to taste.
5. Divide the porridge among bowls and top with your favorite fresh fruit or nuts.

Finished product may be slightly soupy, like cream of wheat.

Oatmeal bake (Serves 6–9)

Ingredients:
- 2 cups old-fashioned rolled oats
- 1 Tbsp. ground flaxseeds
- 2 Tbsp. cinnamon
- 1 tsp. nutmeg
- 1 tsp. baking soda
- 2 large eggs
- 1 1/2 cups of almond milk
- 1/3 cup honey (you may substitute maple syrup or agave nectar)
- 1 cup fresh (or frozen) blueberries
- 2 tsp. vanilla extract
- To drizzle on top: honey, maple syrup or agave nectar

Instructions:
1. Preheat your oven to 375°F. Grease a 9x9 inch baking dish with coconut oil.
2. In a mixing bowl, mix together dry ingredients: rolled oats, ground flaxseeds, cinnamon, nutmeg, and baking soda.
3. In another mixing bowl, whisk together wet ingredients: almond milk, eggs, honey, and vanilla extract.
4. Pour the wet ingredients into the dry ingredients and mix well.

5. Fold in the blueberries and mix until evenly distributed.
6. Pour the mixture into the prepared baking dish and spread it out evenly.
7. Bake for 35–40 minutes, or until the oatmeal bake is golden brown on top and set in the middle.
8. Let it cool for a few minutes before serving.

Drizzle with honey, agave nectar, or maple syrup, if desired.

Oatmeal with pumpkin, pecans, and ground flax seeds (serves 2)

Ingredients:
- 1 cup rolled oats
- 2 cups water
- 1/2 cup canned pumpkin puree
- 1/4 tsp. ground cinnamon
- 1/4 tsp. ground ginger
- 1/8 tsp. ground nutmeg
- 1/8 tsp. salt
- 2 Tbsp. chopped pecans
- 1 Tbsp. ground flax seeds
- 1 Tbsp. honey, maple syrup, or agave nectar (optional)

Instructions:
1. In a medium-sized pot, combine the oats, water, pumpkin puree, cinnamon, ginger, nutmeg, and salt.
2. Bring the mixture to a boil over medium heat.
3. Reduce the heat to low and simmer the oatmeal, stirring occasionally, for 5–7 minutes or until the oats are cooked to your liking.
4. Once the oatmeal is cooked, stir in the chopped pecans and ground flax seeds.

5. Serve the oatmeal hot with a dollop of pumpkin puree. Drizzle with honey, maple syrup or agave nectar if desired.

Almond butter toast with sliced banana and chia seeds (Serves 1)

Ingredients:
- 2 slices of gluten-free bread*
- 2 Tbsp. almond butter
- 1 banana, sliced
- 1/2 tsp. chia seeds
- Dash of cinnamon (optional)
- Drizzle of honey, maple syrup or agave nectar (optional)

Instructions:
1. Toast the bread slices to your desired level of doneness
2. Spread 1 Tbsp. of almond butter on each slice of toast.
3. Arrange the banana slices on top of the almond butter.
4. Sprinkle the chia seeds over the top of the banana slices.
5. Serve immediately and enjoy! You can also add a drizzle of honey, maple syrup or agave nectar and a dash of cinnamon for extra flavor.

*Some gluten-free bread favorites: Udi's, Canyon Bakehouse, Food For Life, Against The Grain.

CHAPTER FOURTEEN
LUNCHES

Chicken and rice bowl (Serves 2)

Ingredients:
- 1 cup uncooked brown rice
- 2 boneless, skinless chicken breasts, cut into 1-inch pieces
- 2 Tbsp. olive oil
- 1 tsp. salt
- 1 tsp. black pepper
- 1 tsp. garlic powder
- 1 tsp. onion powder
- 1 tsp. paprika
- 1 red bell pepper, sliced
- 1 yellow bell pepper, sliced
- 1 small onion, sliced
- 1 avocado, sliced
- 1/4 cup chopped cilantro (optional)
- Lime wedges, for serving (optional)

Instructions:
1. Cook rice according to package instructions.
2. In a large bowl, mix together the chicken, olive oil, salt, pepper, garlic powder, onion powder, and paprika.

3. Heat a large skillet over medium-high heat. Add the chicken and cook until browned; flip halfway through and cook thoroughly, about 6–8 minutes.
4. Add the sliced bell peppers and onion to the skillet and cook until tender, about 5 minutes.
5. To assemble the bowls, divide the cooked rice into 2 bowls. Slice chicken into ½ inch strips. Top rice with the chicken and vegetable mixture. Add sliced avocado. Serve with optional cilantro and lime wedges.

Bibimbap (Serves 2)

Ingredients:

- 1/2 pound beef, sliced into thin strips
- 1/2 cup carrot, julienned
- 1/2 cup zucchini, julienned
- 1/2 cup spinach, blanched and squeezed dry
- 1/2 cup bean sprouts, blanched
- 2 Tbsp. vegetable oil
- 2 Tbsp. soy sauce
- 1 Tbsp. sesame oil
- 1/2 Tbsp. honey
- 2 cloves garlic, minced
- 2 eggs
- Salt and pepper to taste

For the sauce:
- 3 Tbsp. gochujang (Korean red pepper paste)
- 1/2 Tbsp. honey
- 1 Tbsp. sesame oil
- 1 Tbsp. vinegar
- 1 Tbsp. water

Brown rice: follow package instructions.

Instructions:
1. In a small bowl, mix together the soy sauce, sesame oil, honey, and garlic. Add the beef and let it marinate for at least 30 minutes.
2. Heat a large skillet over medium-high heat. Add 1 Tbsp. sesame oil and cook the beef until it's browned and cooked through. Remove from the skillet and set aside in a covered dish to keep warm
3. In the same skillet, add the remaining sesame oil and stir fry the carrots and zucchini for about 2 minutes. Season with salt and pepper to taste. Remove from the skillet and set aside in a covered dish to keep warm.
4. In the same skillet, cook the spinach and bean sprouts until they're heated through. Remove from the skillet and set aside.
5. Fry two eggs in a separate pan in a Tbsp. of sesame seed oil until egg yolks are at preferred consistency.
6. To make the sauce, mix together the gochujang, honey, sesame oil, vinegar, and water in a small bowl. To assemble bibimbap, divide the rice into two bowls. Top each bowl with vegetables, beef, and one fried egg. Drizzle the sauce over top. Stir and enjoy!

Quinoa with chickpeas, spinach, red onion, and tomato
(Serves 4)

Ingredients:
- 1 cup quinoa
- 1 can chickpeas, drained and rinsed
- 1 red onion, diced
- 2 cups fresh spinach, roughly chopped
- 1 cup cherry tomatoes, quartered
- 2 Tbsp. olive oil
- 2 garlic cloves, minced
- 1 tsp. cumin
- 1/2 tsp. salt
- 1/4 tsp. black pepper
- 2 cups vegetable broth

Instructions:
1. Rinse the quinoa in a fine-mesh sieve and place it in a medium saucepan with the vegetable broth. Bring to a boil, then reduce the heat to low and simmer for 15 minutes, or until the quinoa is tender and the liquid has been absorbed. Fluff the quinoa with a fork and set aside.
2. In a large skillet, heat the olive oil over medium-high heat. Add the red onion and cook until it's softened and starting to caramelize, about 5 minutes.

3. Add the garlic, cumin, salt, and pepper to the skillet. Cook for 1–2 minutes, or until fragrant.
4. Add the chickpeas to the skillet. Cook for 2–3 minutes, or until heated through.
5. Add the spinach to the skillet and cook until wilted, about 2 minutes.
6. Add the tomato to the skillet and cook for 1–2 minutes, or until softened.
7. Add the cooked quinoa to the skillet and stir everything together until well combined.
8. Serve hot and enjoy!

You can also customize this recipe by adding other veggies or spices that you like, such as roasted bell peppers, zucchini, or smoked paprika. It is a versatile vegan dish that can be served alone or as a side dish with chicken, beef, or fish. Can also be served chilled.

Lentil soup (Serves 6)

Lentils are my favorite vegan protein. This soup is my favorite all year round. Double the batch if you would like to freeze some for later.

Ingredients:
- 1 cup green lentils, rinsed and drained
- 6 cups vegetable broth
- 1 cup carrots, chopped
- 1 cup celery, chopped
- 1/2 cup yellow onion, chopped
- 2 cloves garlic
- 1 tsp. ground cumin
- 1 tsp. smoked paprika
- 2 Tbsp. olive oil
- 2 bay leaves
- 2 Tbsp. thyme
- Salt and pepper, to taste
- Juice of 1/2 lemon
- Chopped fresh parsley, for garnish

Instructions:
1. Heat the olive oil in a large pot over medium heat. Add carrots, celery, onion and garlic, and cook until softened, about 5–7 minutes.

2. Add the ground cumin and smoked paprika to the vegetable mixture, and cook for another minute, stirring constantly.
3. Add the green lentils, vegetable broth, and bay leaves to the pot. Bring the soup to a boil, then reduce the heat and let it simmer for 30–40 minutes, or until the lentils are tender.
4. Remove the bay leaves from the soup and discard. Season the soup with salt and pepper, to taste.
5. Put 1 cup of finished soup into a medium bowl. Use an immersion blender and blend until smooth. Add this cup of soup back into the pot of soup for a creamier consistency.
6. Stir in the lemon juice and adjust the seasoning, if needed.
7. Serve the soup hot, garnished with chopped fresh parsley.

Green salad with baked chicken (Serves 2)

Ingredients:
- 2 boneless, skinless chicken breasts
- 1 Tbsp. olive oil
- 1/2 tsp. salt
- 1/4 tsp. black pepper
- 1/4 tsp. garlic powder
- 4 cups mixed greens (such as romaine lettuce, arugula, spinach)
- 1/2 cucumber, sliced
- 1/2 cup cherry tomatoes, halved
- 1/4 cup sliced red onion
- 1 avocado, sliced
- Simple vinaigrette dressing (page 183)

Instructions:
1. Preheat the oven to 400°F. Place the chicken breasts in a baking dish and drizzle with olive oil. Season with salt, pepper, and garlic powder
2. Roast the chicken in the oven for 20–25 minutes or until the internal temperature reaches 165°F.
3. Remove the chicken from the oven and let it rest for 5 minutes. Slice the chicken into ½ inch strips.
4. In a large bowl, toss the mixed greens with the cucumber, avocado, cherry tomatoes, and red onion.
5. Add the sliced chicken to the salad.

6. Top with sliced avocado
7. Drizzle with simple vinaigrette and toss to combine.
8. Serve the salad immediately and enjoy!

Roasted veggies with tempeh over rice (serves 2)

Ingredients:
- 1 large sweet potato, peeled and chopped into bite-size pieces
- 2 cups Brussels sprouts, halved
- 2 cups sliced mushrooms (cremini or baby portabello)
- 1/2 red onion, chopped
- 1 Tbsp. olive oil
- Salt and pepper, to taste
- 8 oz. tempeh, sliced*

Brown rice: follow instructions on the package

Instructions:
1. Preheat the oven to 400°F.
2. In a large bowl, toss the sweet potato, Brussels sprouts, mushrooms, and red onion with olive oil. Season with salt and pepper.
3. Spread the vegetables out on a baking sheet and roast in the oven for 25–30 minutes, stirring occasionally, until the vegetables are tender and slightly browned.
4. While the vegetables are roasting, cook the rice according to package directions.
5. In a large skillet, sauté the tempeh over medium-high heat until it is lightly browned.

6. Once the vegetables are done roasting, add them to the skillet with the seitan and stir to combine.
7. Serve the seitan and vegetable mixture over the rice and enjoy!

Note: You can customize this dish by adding your favorite vegetables, and also by adding additional seasonings (such as garlic or rosemary) for added flavor.

*Tempeh, which is a fermented soy product, can be an acquired taste, but I felt compelled to add it to the recipes as it is a wonderful vegan protein. If you do not like tempeh at all, substitute baked chicken, like the one presented in the recipe before this one on page 155.

Grilled tofu bowl with tahini dressing (Serves 2)

Ingredients:

For the Grilled Tofu:
- 1 block of firm tofu, pressed and drained
- 2 Tbsp. of tamari *
- 1 Tbsp. of maple syrup
- 1 Tbsp. of olive oil
- 1 clove of garlic, minced
- Salt and pepper, to taste

For the Bowl:
- 1 sliced avocado
- ½ sliced cucumber
- 1 sliced bell pepper
- 1 sliced carrot
- ½ sliced red onion
- Herbs such as cilantro, parsley (optional)

Brown rice or quinoa: follow package instructions

Instructions:
1. Preheat an iron skillet or heavy Dutch oven to medium-high heat.
2. Cut the tofu into cubes or slices.
3. In a small bowl, whisk together tamari, maple syrup, olive oil, garlic, salt, and pepper.

4. Place the tofu in a shallow dish and pour the marinade over it, tossing to coat.
5. Grill the tofu for about 5-7 minutes on each side, until nicely charred. Pour remaining tamari and maple syrup mixture over tofu while cooking.
6. Assemble the bowls, placing one cup of cooked quinoa or brown rice into four bowls. Top with grilled tofu, sliced avocado, cucumber, bell pepper, carrot, and red onion.
7. Top with a few dashes of tamari to taste.

*Tamari is a gluten-free substitute for soy sauce, found in the Asian food aisle at any supermarket.

Beet and chicken salad (Serves 2)

Ingredients:
- 2 boneless, skinless chicken breasts
- 4 cups arugula
- 1/2 cup pumpkin seeds
- 2 Tbsp. olive oil
- Garlic powder
- Salt and pepper to taste
- Roasted beets (page 188)
- Tangy orange dressing (page 182) *

Instructions:
1. Preheat your oven to 400°F.
2. Make roasted beets from instructions on page 188. While the beets are roasting, rub olive oil onto chicken and season with garlic powder, salt, and pepper, and roast them in the oven for about 20–25 minutes, or until they are cooked through. Let the chicken cool slightly before slicing into ½ inch slices.
3. Toast the pumpkin seeds in a dry skillet over medium heat, stirring frequently, until they are lightly browned and fragrant.
4. Arrange arugula on two plates and top with sliced chicken, roasted beets, and pumpkin seeds. Drizzle the dressing over the salad and serve immediately.

*You may substitute simple vinaigrette from page 183 if you'd like.

Quinoa with arugula, sweet potatoes, and pomegranate
(Serves 2)

Ingredients:
- 1 cup quinoa, rinsed and drained
- 2 cups water
- 2 cups arugula, washed and dried
- 1/2 cup pomegranate seeds
- 1/4 cup pine nuts (optional)
- Roasted sweet potatoes (page 189)
- Honey dijon mustard dressing (page 184)

Instructions:
1. In a medium saucepan, combine the quinoa and water. Bring to a boil, reduce heat to low, and simmer, covered, for 15–20 minutes or until the water is absorbed and the quinoa is tender. Fluff with a fork and set aside.
2. In a large bowl, mix the roasted sweet potatoes, arugula, pomegranate, and optional pine nuts.
3. Divide quinoa into two bowls and serve sweet potato, arugula, pomegranate, and optional pine nut mixture on top.
4. Drizzle with dressing and enjoy!
5. Can be served warm or chilled. Can also be served as a side dish with chicken, beef, fish, or grilled tofu.

CHAPTER FIFTEEN
DINNERS

Baked salmon with asparagus and cauliflower mash
(Serves 2)

Ingredients:
- 2 salmon filets
- 2 lemons, sliced
- 1 Tbsp. olive oil
- Salt and pepper, to taste
- Steamed asparagus (page 190)
- Cauliflower mash (page 186)
- Parsley sauce (page 184)

Instructions:
1. Preheat the oven to 375°.
2. Slice the lemons into 1/4 inch slices and place in one layer in the bottom of a baking dish.
3. Place the salmon filets, skin down, on the lemon slices.
4. Brush salmon filets with olive oil.
5. Bake in the oven for 15–20 minutes, or until the salmon is cooked through and flakes easily with a fork.
6. Serve the salmon with cauliflower mash and steamed asparagus. Drizzle with parsley sauce.

Baked chicken with sweet and tart spinach (Serves 2)

Ingredients:
- 2 boneless, skinless chicken breasts
- 2 Tbsp. olive oil
- 1 tsp. garlic powder
- 1 tsp. onion powder
- 1 tsp. paprika
- 1/2 tsp. dried thyme
- Salt and pepper to taste
- Sweet and tart spinach (page 191)

Instructions:
1. Preheat oven to 400°F.
2. Lightly grease a baking dish with avocado oil.
3. In a small bowl, mix together olive oil, garlic powder, onion powder, paprika, dried thyme, salt, and pepper.
4. Rub the mixture onto both sides of the chicken breasts.
5. Place the chicken breasts in the baking dish and bake for 22–25 minutes, or until the chicken is cooked through and the juices run clear.
6. Once done, remove the chicken from the oven and let it rest for a few minutes before slicing and serving with a side of sweet and tart spinach.

Beef stew (Serves 4)

Ingredients:
- 2 pounds beef chuck, cut into 1-inch pieces
- 3 Tbsp. all-purpose flour
- 2 Tbsp. vegetable oil
- 1 large onion, chopped
- 2 cloves garlic, minced
- 4 cups beef broth
- 2 cups water
- 1 tsp. salt
- 1/2 tsp. black pepper
- 1/2 tsp. dried thyme
- 2 bay leaves
- 4 carrots, peeled and cut into 1-inch pieces
- 3 Yukon Gold potatoes, peeled and cut into 1-inch pieces
- 1 cup frozen peas
- Chopped fresh parsley for garnish

Instructions:
1. In a large bowl, toss the beef with the flour until well-coated.
2. In a Dutch oven or large pot, heat the oil over medium-high heat. Add the beef and cook until browned on all sides, about 5–7 minutes.
3. Add the onion and garlic and cook for 2–3 minutes until softened.

4. Add the beef broth, water, salt, pepper, thyme, and bay leaves. Bring to a simmer, then reduce the heat to low and cover the pot. Cook for 1 1/2 to 2 hours, stirring occasionally, until the beef is tender.
5. Add the carrots and potatoes to the pot and continue cooking for an additional 30–40 minutes, until the vegetables are tender.
6. Add the frozen peas to the pot and cook for an additional 5–10 minutes.
7. Remove the bay leaves and discard. Taste the stew and adjust the seasoning if necessary.
8. Serve hot, garnished with chopped fresh parsley. Enjoy!

Note: If you prefer a thicker stew, whisk a teaspoon of white flour with cold water to make a slurry. Slowly add slurry into the stew while stirring. Avoid adding dry flour directly to stew, as flour can clump.

Tofu stir fry with brown rice (Serves 2)

Ingredients:
- 1 block of firm tofu
- 2 Tbsp. sesame oil
- 2 cloves of garlic, minced
- 2 Tbsp. grated ginger
- 3 sliced carrots
- 3 sliced celery stalks
- 1/2 cup water chestnuts
- 2 Tbsp. tamari sauce
- Salt and pepper to taste

Serve over brown rice. To cook brown rice, follow instructions on the package.

Instructions:
1. Press the tofu to remove any excess water. Cut it into 1-inch cubes and set aside.
2. Heat the oil in a large skillet or wok over medium-high heat.
3. Add the garlic and ginger to the skillet and cook for 1–2 minutes until fragrant.
4. Add the celery and carrots to the skillet and stir fry for 3–4 minutes until the vegetables are tender.
5. Add the tofu to the skillet and stir fry for 2–3 minutes until the tofu is slightly browned.

6. Pour the tamari sauce over the tofu and vegetables and stir to combine.
7. Season with salt and pepper to taste.
8. Serve the tofu stir fry over the cooked brown rice. Drizzle with more tamari sauce, if desired.

Quinoa with arugula, sweet potato, avocado, and eggs (Serves 2)

Ingredients:
- 1 cup quinoa
- 2 cups water
- 2 Tbsp. olive oil
- Salt and pepper, to taste
- 2 cups arugula
- 1 avocado, sliced
- 4 eggs
- Black sesame seeds
- Balsamic glaze

Roasted sweet potatoes (page 189)

Instructions:
1. Rinse the quinoa in a fine-mesh strainer under running water. In a medium-sized pot, add the quinoa and water and bring to a boil. Reduce the heat to low, cover, and simmer for 15 minutes.
2. While the quinoa is cooking, prepare roasted sweet potatoes from page 189.
3. In a separate, non-stick skillet, cook the eggs in olive oil to your desired doneness.
4. When the quinoa is done cooking, fluff it with a fork and divide it into two bowls. Top each bowl

with the sweet potato, arugula, avocado, and a cooked egg.
5. Top with a dash of black sesame seeds and enjoy!

Optional: Serve over brown rice instead of quinoa, if preferred. You can also add a drizzle of balsamic glaze to add an additional, complementary flavor to the dish.

Pan-seared steak salad (Serves 2)

Ingredients:
- 1 New York strip steak
- Tamara's marinade (page 185)
- 1 Tbsp. olive oil
- 4 cups mixed salad greens
- 3/4 cup cherry tomatoes, halved
- 1/2 cup sliced red, yellow, and orange bell peppers
- Honey Dijon mustard dressing (page 184)

Instructions:
1. Place steak in a covered dish with Tamara's marinade and rest for as little as 30 minutes or as long as overnight.
2. Remove steak from the refrigerator. Pat dry, then let it sit at room temperature for 20–30 minutes. Preheat an iron skillet or Dutch oven over high heat.
3. Put 1 tablespoon of olive oil into a heated skillet, then place steak and sear for 4–5 minutes on each side or until the desired level of doneness is reached. Turn the steak on its sides to brown for an additional 2-3 minutes Check doneness by making a small cut with a steak knife into the center. Remove the steak from the skillet and let it rest for 10 minutes.

4. While the steak is resting, assemble the salad. In a large bowl, combine the salad greens, cherry tomatoes, and sliced peppers.
5. Once the steak has rested, slice it into 1-inch strips against the grain.
6. Divide salad onto two plates, add the sliced steak to the salad, and drizzle the dressing on top.
7. Serve the salad immediately and enjoy!

Lamb stew with dates and sweet potatoes (Serves 4)

Ingredients:
- 1 1/2 lb. lamb stew meat, cut into bite-size pieces
- 2 Tbsp. olive oil
- 1 onion, diced
- 2 cloves garlic, minced
- 2 tsp. ground cumin
- 1 tsp. ground coriander
- 1/2 tsp. ground cinnamon
- 1/2 tsp. ground ginger
- 1/4 tsp. cayenne pepper (optional)
- 3 cups low-sodium chicken broth
- 2 medium sweet potatoes, peeled and cut into 1-inch cubes
- 1 cup pitted dates, chopped
- Salt and pepper, to taste
- Chopped fresh cilantro, for garnish (optional)

Directions:

1. Heat olive oil in a large pot over medium-high heat. Add lamb and cook until browned on all sides, about 5 minutes. Remove lamb from the pot and set aside.
2. Add onion to the same pot and cook until softened, about 3 minutes. Add garlic, cumin, coriander,

cinnamon, ginger, and cayenne pepper (if using) and cook for 1 minute more.

3. Add chicken broth and bring to a simmer, scraping any browned bits from the bottom of the pot. Add sweet potatoes and dates. Return lamb to the pot. Bring to a boil, then reduce heat and simmer, covered, until lamb is tender and sweet potatoes are cooked through, about 45 minutes.

4. Season with salt and pepper to taste. Serve hot. Garnish with chopped cilantro (optional).

Note: If you prefer a thicker stew, whisk a teaspoon of white flour with cold water to make a slurry. Slowly add slurry into the stew while stirring. Avoid adding dry flour directly to stew, as flour can clump.

Pan-seared steak with portobello mushrooms and zucchini (Serves 1)

Ingredients:
- 1 New York strip steak
- 1 Tbsp. olive oil
- Tamara's marinade (page 185)
- Roasted portobello mushrooms and zucchini (page 187)

Instructions:
1. Place steak in a covered dish with Tamara's marinade and rest for as little as 30 minutes or as long as overnight.
2. Remove steak from the refrigerator, pat dry and let it sit at room temperature for 20–30 minutes. Preheat an iron skillet or Dutch oven over high heat.
3. Put 1 tablespoon of olive oil into a heated skillet, then place steak and sear for 4–5 minutes on each side or until the desired level of doneness is reached. Turn the steak on its sides to brown for an additional 2-3 minutes. Check doneness by making a small cut with a steak knife into the center. Remove the steak from the skillet and let it rest for 10 minutes.
4. Serve with roasted portobello mushrooms and zucchini and enjoy!

Veggie stir fry with almonds (Serves 2)

Ingredients:
- 2 Tbsp. avocado oil
- 1 onion, sliced
- 3 cloves garlic, minced
- 1 Tbsp. ginger, minced
- 1 red bell pepper, sliced
- 1 green bell pepper, sliced
- 1 cup sliced mushrooms
- 1 cup snow peas
- 2/3 cup slivered almonds
- 2 Tbsp. tamari sauce
- 1 tsp. sesame oil
- Salt and pepper, to taste

Brown rice. Follow package instructions.

Instructions:
1. Prepare brown rice with instructions on the package.
2. While rice is cooking, heat the sesame oil in a wok or large skillet over high heat.
3. Add the onion, garlic and ginger, and stir fry for 1–2 minutes until fragrant.
4. Add the red and green bell peppers, mushrooms, and snow peas, and stir fry for another 3–4 minutes until the vegetables are tender-crisp.

5. Add the slivered almonds and continue to stir fry for another 1–2 minutes until the almonds are toasted and fragrant.
6. In a small bowl, whisk together the tamari sauce, sesame oil, salt, and pepper.
7. Pour the sauce over the stir fry and toss to coat.
8. Serve hot over brown rice and enjoy!

CHAPTER SIXTEEN
SAUCES, DRESSINGS, AND SIDE DISHES

I think this is my favorite part of the entire recipe portion of this book. A good sauce or dressing can turn a simple meal into something extraordinary. You will need a high speed blender or a small whisk and bowl to prepare the following dressings and sauces. You can store them in an airtight container in the refrigerator for up to one week.

SAUCES AND DRESSINGS

Tahini dressing

- 1/4 cup tahini
- 1/4 cup water
- 2 Tbsp. lemon juice
- 1 clove garlic, minced
- 1/2 tsp. salt
- 1/4 tsp. black pepper

Instructions:
1. In a small bowl, whisk together the tahini and water until smooth.
2. Add lemon juice, minced garlic, salt, and black pepper. Whisk until everything is combined.

3. If the dressing is too thick, add more water, 1 tablespoon at a time, until it reaches your desired consistency.
4. Taste the dressing and adjust the seasoning as needed. If you prefer a tangier dressing, add more lemon juice, and if you like a spicier dressing, add a pinch of cayenne pepper.
5. Serve the tahini dressing immediately or store it in an airtight container in the refrigerator for up to a week.

Tangy orange dressing

- 1/4 cup freshly squeezed orange juice
- 1/4 cup extra-virgin olive oil
- 1 Tbsp. honey
- 1 Tbsp. Dijon mustard
- Salt and pepper to taste

Instructions:
1. In a small bowl, whisk together the orange juice, honey, Dijon mustard, salt, and pepper.
2. Slowly drizzle in the olive oil, whisking constantly, until the dressing is emulsified.
3. Taste the dressing and adjust the seasoning as needed.

4. Serve the dressing immediately or store it in an airtight container in the refrigerator for up to one week.
5. Give the dressing a good shake or whisk before using it again, as the oil and juice may separate while in the refrigerator.

Simple vinaigrette dressing

- 1/4 cup balsamic vinegar
- 1/2 cup extra virgin olive oil
- 1 clove garlic, minced (optional)
- 1 tsp. honey
- Salt and pepper, to taste

Instructions:

1. In a small bowl, whisk together the balsamic vinegar, minced garlic, honey, salt, and pepper until combined.
2. Slowly drizzle in the olive oil while whisking continuously to emulsify the mixture.
3. Keep whisking until the dressing is well blended and slightly thickened.
4. Taste and adjust the seasoning as desired.
5. Serve immediately over your favorite salad or store in an airtight container in the refrigerator for up to one week.

Parsley sauce

- 1/4 cup parsley
- 1/4 cup olive oil
- 1 tsp. minced garlic
- Salt and pepper

1. Finely chop parsley.
2. Whisk parsley, olive oil, and garlic in a bowl. Add salt and pepper to taste. Serve over meat, fish, or vegetables.

Honey dijon dressing

- 1/8 cup Dijon mustard
- 1/8 cup honey
- 1/8 cup apple cider vinegar
- 1/4 cup olive oil
- Salt and pepper to taste

Instructions:

1. In a medium-sized mixing bowl, whisk together the Dijon mustard, honey, and apple cider vinegar until well combined.

2. Slowly pour in the olive oil, whisking constantly to emulsify the dressing. This will create a smooth and creamy consistency.
3. Add salt and pepper to taste and continue whisking until fully incorporated.

Tamara's marinade

- 1/4 cup balsamic vinegar
- 1/4 cup soy sauce
- 1/4 cup Worcestershire sauce
- 1 Tbsp. minced garlic
- 2 Tbsp. olive oil

Whisk all ingredients together in a glass dish.

SIDE DISHES

Cauliflower mash

Cauliflower mash is very simple to prepare and can take the place of mashed potatoes—which is a great solution if you are watching carbohydrate intake.

Ingredients:

- 1 head of cauliflower
- 2 garlic cloves, minced
- 2 Tbsp. of vegan butter (Earth Balance, Kite Hill, or Miyoko's)
- 1/4 cup of unsweetened almond milk (or other non-dairy milk)
- Salt and pepper to taste

Instructions:
1. Cut the cauliflower into small florets and rinse them well.
2. Bring a large pot of salted water to a boil. Add the cauliflower florets and garlic to the pot and boil for 10–15 minutes, or until the cauliflower is soft.
3. Drain the water and transfer the cauliflower and garlic to a food processor or blender. Add vegan butter, almond milk, and salt and pepper to taste.

4. Pulse or puree the mixture until it is your desired smoothness and creaminess. You may need to stop and scrape down the sides of the food processor or blender a few times during mixing.
5. Taste cauliflower mash and adjust the seasoning as needed.
6. Serve hot and enjoy!

Roasted portobello mushrooms and zucchini

Ingredients:

- 2 large portobello mushrooms, stems removed
- 2 medium zucchini, sliced
- 3 cloves of garlic, minced
- 3 Tbsp. of olive oil
- 1 Tbsp. of balsamic vinegar
- Salt and pepper, to taste

Instructions:
1. Preheat your oven to 400°F.
2. Clean the portobello mushrooms with a damp paper towel and remove the stems. Slice them into thick pieces.
3. Slice the zucchini into rounds or half-moons, about 1/4 inch thick.

4. In a large mixing bowl, combine the sliced mushrooms and zucchini. Add olive oil and minced garlic to the vegetables and toss to coat evenly.
5. Spread the vegetables out in a single layer on a baking sheet lined with parchment paper. Add salt and pepper to taste.
6. Roast the vegetables in the oven for 20–25 minutes, until the zucchini is tender and the mushrooms are cooked through.

Roasted beets

Ingredients:
- 2 medium-sized beets
- 2 Tbsp. olive oil
- Salt and pepper, to taste

Instructions:
1. Preheat your oven to 375°F.
2. Scrub the beets under running water to remove any dirt.
3. Cut off the greens and the tails of the beets. Peel off the skin using a vegetable peeler.
4. Cut the beets into cubes, or slice them into wedges or rounds, whichever you prefer.
5. Toss the beets in a bowl with the olive oil, salt, and pepper until the beets are evenly coated.

6. Spread the beets in a single layer on a baking sheet or a roasting pan.
7. Roast the beets in the preheated oven for 30 to 40 minutes, or until they are tender and caramelized. Flip the beets halfway through the cooking time to ensure even cooking.
8. Once the beets are done, remove them from the oven and let them cool for a few minutes before serving.

Roasted sweet potatoes

Ingredients:

- 2 large sweet potatoes, peeled and diced into 1-inch cubes
- 2 Tbsp. olive oil
- Salt and pepper to taste

Instructions:
1. Preheat the oven to 400°.
2. Peel the sweet potatoes and dice them into 1-inch cubes.
3. In a large mixing bowl, toss the sweet potato cubes with olive oil, salt, and pepper. Make sure the sweet potatoes are evenly coated with oil.
4. Spread the sweet potato cubes out on a baking sheet in a single layer.

5. Roast the sweet potatoes in the preheated oven for 25–30 minutes, or until they are tender and golden brown. You can use a spatula to stir the sweet potatoes halfway through the cooking time to ensure they cook evenly.
6. Remove the sweet potatoes from the oven and let them cool for a few minutes before serving.

Steamed asparagus

Ingredients:

- 1 pound asparagus, woody ends trimmed off
- 2 cloves garlic, minced
- 2 Tbsp. olive oil
- 1/2 tsp. salt
- 1/4 tsp. black pepper

Instructions:
1. Rinse the asparagus under cold water and trim off the woody ends, about 1 inch from the bottom
2. In a large pot or a steamer basket, bring 1–2 inches of water to a boil over medium-high heat.
3. Once the water is boiling, place the asparagus in the steamer basket, cover with a lid, and steam for 5–7 minutes, or until the asparagus is tender.

4. While the asparagus is steaming, heat the olive oil in a small skillet over medium heat. Add the minced garlic and cook for 1–2 minutes, or until fragrant and slightly golden.
5. Once the asparagus is cooked, remove it from the steamer basket and place it in a serving dish.
6. Drizzle the garlic-infused olive oil over the asparagus. Add salt and pepper.
7. Toss the asparagus gently to ensure that it is evenly coated with the garlic oil and seasoning.
8. Serve hot and enjoy!

Sweet and Tart Spinach

Ingredients:

- 2 cups fresh spinach leaves, washed and coarsely chopped
- 1 green apple, cored and diced
- 1/4 cup chopped walnuts
- 2 Tbsp. olive oil
- 1 Tbsp. apple cider vinegar
- 1 Tbsp. honey or agave nectar
- Salt and pepper, to taste

Instructions:

1. In a large bowl, combine the chopped spinach, diced apple, and chopped walnuts.
2. In a separate small bowl, whisk together the olive oil, apple cider vinegar, honey or agave nectar, and a pinch of salt and pepper.
3. Pour the dressing over the spinach and apple mixture, and toss to combine.
4. Add additional salt and pepper to taste.
5. Serve the spinach and green apple salad immediately as a side dish.

NOTES

INTRODUCTION

1. Maltz, M. *Psycho-Cybernetics*. London: Churchill Livingstone, 1960.

SECTION ONE-THE FORBIDDENS

CHAPTER ONE-SUGAR

1. Goran MI, Plows JF, Ventura EE. "Effects of consuming sugars and alternative sweeteners during pregnancy on maternal and child health: evidence for a secondhand sugar effect." *Proceedings of the Nutrition Society.* (2019 Aug);78(3):262-271.
2. Hatch EE, Wesselink AK, Hahn KA, Michiel JJ, Mikkelsen EM, Sorensen HT, Rothman KJ, Wise LA. "Intake of sugar-sweetened beverages and fecundability in a North American preconception cohort." *Epidemiology.* (2018 May);29(3):369-378.
3. Willis, Sydney K., Lauren A. Wise, Amelia K. Wesselink, Kenneth J. Rothman, Ellen M. Mikkelsen, Katherine L. Tucker, Ellen Trolle, and Elizabeth E. Hatch. "Glycemic load, dietary fiber, and added sugar and fecundability in 2 preconception cohorts." *The American Journal of Clinical Nutrition.* (July 1, 2020); 112, no. 1:27–38.

CHAPTER TWO-CAFFEINE

1. American College of Obstetricians and Gynecologists. (2020). Nutrition during pregnancy. Retrieved from https://www.acog.org/womens-health/faqs/nutrition-during-pregnancy
2. James, JE. "Maternal caffeine consumption and pregnancy outcomes: a narrative review with implications for advice to mothers and mothers-to-be." *BMJ Evidence-Based Medicine.* (2021);26:114-115.
3. Weng X, Odouli R, Li DK. "Maternal caffeine consumption during pregnancy and the risk of miscarriage: a prospective cohort study." *American Journal of Obstetrics and Gynecology.* (2008);198(3):279.e1-8.
4. Jin, F., Qiao, C. "Association of maternal caffeine intake during pregnancy with low birth weight, childhood overweight, and obesity: a meta-analysis of cohort studies." *International Journal of Obesity.* (2021);45, 279–287.

CHAPTER THREE-ALCOHOL

1. Fan, D., Liu, L., Xia, Q. *et al.* "Female alcohol consumption and fecundability: a systematic review and dose-response meta-analysis." *Scientific Reports.* (2017);7, 13815.
2. Centers for Disease Control and Prevention. "Alcohol use in pregnancy." https://www.cdc.gov/ncbddd/fasd/alcohol-use.html. Accessed February 17, 2023.

3. Sayal K, Heron J, Golding J, et al. "Binge pattern of alcohol consumption during pregnancy and childhood mental health outcomes: longitudinal population-based study." *Pediatrics*. (2009);123(2): e289-296.
4. O'Leary CM, Nassar N, Kurinczuk JJ, et al. "Prenatal alcohol exposure and risk of birth defects." *Pediatrics*. (2010);126(4): e843-850.

CHAPTER FOUR-ICED/COLD/FROZEN FOOD AND BEVERAGES

1. Maciocia, Giovanni. *Obstetrics and Gynecology in Chinese Medicine*. London: Churchill Livingstone, 2011.
2. Pitchford, Paul. *Healing with Whole Foods: Asian Traditions and Modern Nutrition*. Berkeley: North Atlantic Books, 2002.

SECTION TWO-LIFESTYLE

1. Sharma, M., & Rush, S. E. "Mindfulness-Based Stress Reduction as a Stress Management Intervention for Healthy Individuals: A Systematic Review." *Journal of Evidence-Based Complementary & Alternative Medicine*, (2014):19(4), 271-286.
2. Newsom, R. "Relaxation Exercises to Help Fall Asleep," *National Sleep Foundation*. (April 1, 2022). https://www.sleepfoundation.org/relaxation

CHAPTER FIVE-SLEEP

1. Lateef OM, Akintubosun MO. "Sleep and reproductive health." *Journal of Circadian Rhythms.* (2020 Mar);23;18:1.
2. Beroukhim, G., Esencan, E., Seifer, D. B., "Impact of sleep patterns upon female neuroendocrinology and reproductive outcomes: a comprehensive review." *Reproductive Biology and Endocrinology* 20, 16 (2022). https://rbej.biomedcentral.com/articles/10.1186/s12958-022-00889-3
3. Okun ML, Schetter CD, Glynn LM. Poor sleep quality is associated with preterm birth. *Sleep.* (2011 Nov 1);34(11):1493-8.
4. Kloss JD, Perlis ML, Zamzow JA, Culnan EJ, Gracia CR. "Sleep, sleep disturbance, and fertility in women." *Sleep Medicine Reviews.* (2015 Aug);22:78-87.

CHAPTER SIX-ACUPUNCTURE

1. Zhong Y, Zeng F, Liu W, Ma J, Guan Y, Song Y. (2019). "Acupuncture in improving endometrial receptivity: a systematic review and meta-analysis." *Reproductive Biology and Endocrinology.* (2019 Mar 13);19(1):61.
2. Wu, Jm., Ning, Y., Ye, Yy. *et al.* "Effects of acupuncture on endometrium and pregnancy outcomes in patients with polycystic ovarian syndrome undergoing

in vitro fertilization-embryo transfer: a randomized clinical trial." *Chinese Journal of Integrative Medicine.* (2022);28;736–742.
3. Diogo Amorim, Irma Brito, Armando Caseiro, João Paulo Figueiredo, André Pinto, Inês Macedo, Jorge Machado. "Electroacupuncture and acupuncture in the treatment of anxiety - A double blinded randomized parallel clinical trial." *Complementary Therapies in Clinical Practice.* Volume 46, (2022); 101541, ISSN 1744-3881.
4. Setiawardhani, A. L., A. Srilestari, and C. Simadibrata. "Electroacupuncture effect at the LI 4 Hegu point on the plasma β-endorphin level of healthy subjects." *Journal of Physics: Conference Series.* (2017);vol. 884, no. 1, p. 012027.

CHAPTER SEVEN-EXERCISE

1. Aria, Behzad, Amin Salegi-abarghui, Mohammad Hasan Lotfi, and Masoud Mirzaei. "Effect of exercise, body mass index, and waist to hip ratio on female fertility." *Journal of Basic Research in Medical Science.* 7, no. 3 (2020); 19-25.
2. Xie F, You Y, Guan C, Gu Y, Yao F, Xu J. "Association between physical activity and infertility: a comprehensive systematic review and meta-analysis." *Journal of Translational Medicine.* (2022 May 23);20(1):237.
3. Hakimi, O., Cameron, LC. "Effect of Exercise on Ovulation: A Systematic Review." *Sports Medicine.* (2017);47, 1555–1567 .

CHAPTER EIGHT-SUPPLEMENTS

1. Mayo Clinic. (2021). "Prenatal vitamins: Why they matter, how to choose." Retrieved from https://www.mayoclinic.org/healthy-lifestyle/pregnancy-week-by-week/in-depth/prenatal-vitamins/art-20046945
2. American College of Obstetricians and Gynecologists. (2021). Nutrition during pregnancy. Retrieved from https://www.acog.org/womens-health/faqs/nutrition-during-pregnancy

CHAPTER NINE-PRENATAL VITAMINS

1. American College of Obstetricians and Gynecologists. (2021). Nutrition during pregnancy. Retrieved from https://www.acog.org/womens-health/faqs/nutrition-during-pregnancy
2. https://americanpregnancy.org/healthy-pregnancy/pregnancy-health-wellness/types-prenatal-vitamins/

CHAPTER TEN-COENZYME Q10 (COQ10)

1. Ben-Meir, A., Burstein, E., Borrego-Alvarez, A., Chong, J., Wong, E., Yavorska, T., ... & Jurisicova, A. "Coenzyme Q10 restores oocyte mitochondrial function and fertility during reproductive aging." *Aging cell*. (2015);14(5):887-95.

2. Zhang D, Keilty D, Zhang ZF, Chian RC. "Mitochondria in oocyte aging: current understanding." *Facts, Views & Visions in ObGyn.* (2017 Mar);9(1):29-38.
3. Florou P, Anagnostis P, Theocharis P, Chourdakis M, Goulis DG. "Does coenzyme Q10 supplementation improve fertility outcomes in women undergoing assisted reproductive technology procedures? A systematic review and meta-analysis of randomized-controlled trials." *Journal of Assisted Reproduction and Genetics.* (2020 Oct);37(10):2377-2387.
4. Xu Y, Nisenblat V, Lu C, Li R, Qiao J, Zhen X, Wang S. "Pretreatment with coenzyme Q10 improves ovarian response and embryo quality in low-prognosis young women with decreased ovarian reserve: a randomized controlled trial." *Reproductive Biology and Endocrinology.* (2018 Mar 27);16(1):29.
5. Alahmar AT. The impact of two doses of coenzyme Q10 on semen parameters and antioxidant status in men with idiopathic oligoasthenoteratozoospermia. *Clinical and Experimental Reproductive Medicine.* (2019 Sep);46(3):112-118.
6. Cleveland Clinic. "Heart Problems During Pregnancy," n.d. https://my.clevelandclinic.org/health/diseases/17068-heart-disease--pregnancy#:~:text=Cardiovascular%20disease%20is%20a%20leading,conditions%20like%20high%20blood%20pressure.

CHAPTER ELEVEN-VITAMIN D3

1. "Nutrition During Pregnancy."
2. Xu F, Wolf S, Green O, Xu J. "Vitamin D in follicular development and oocyte maturation." *Reproduction.* (2021 May 5);161(6):R129-R137.
3. Zhao J, Liu S, Wang Y, et al. "Vitamin D improves in-vitro fertilization outcomes in infertile women with polycystic ovary syndrome and insulin resistance." *Minerva Medica.* (2019 Jun);110(3):199-208.
4. Tripkovic L, Lambert H, Hart K, et al. "Comparison of vitamin D2 and vitamin D3 supplementation in raising serum 25-hydroxyvitamin D status: a systematic review and meta-analysis." *American Journal of Clinical Nutrition.* (2012);95(6):1357-1364.

CHAPTER TWELVE-THE PLAN!

1. Caut, Cherie, Matthew Leach, and Amie Steel. "Dietary guideline adherence during preconception and pregnancy: A systematic review." *Maternal & Child Nutrition* 16, no. 2 (2020); e12916.
2. https://www.dietaryguidelines.gov/sites/default/files/2021-03/Dietary_Guidelines_for_Americans-2020-2025.pdf (pg. 107-118)
3. Pitchford
4. Kim K, Wactawski-Wende J, Michels KA, Plowden TC, Chaljub EN, Sjaarda LA, Mumford SL. "Dairy Food Intake

Is Associated with Reproductive Hormones and Sporadic Anovulation among Healthy Premenopausal Women." *The Journal of Nutrition.* (2017 Feb);147(2):218-226.

5. Chavarro JE, Rich-Edwards JW, Rosner B, Willett WC. "A prospective study of dairy foods intake and anovulatory infertility." *Human Reproduction.* (2007 May);22(5):1340-7.
6. Maciocia, G. *Obstetrics and Gynecology in Chinese Medicine* (2nd ed.). London: Churchill Livingstone, 2011.
7. Bold, Justine & Diamantopoulou, Dimitra. "Views and experiences of infertile women regarding the role of gluten in their infertility." *Obstetrics and Gynecology Research.* (2022);05. 10.26502/ogr0104.
8. Unanue W, Gomez Mella ME, Cortez DA, Bravo D, Araya-Véliz C, Unanue J, Van Den Broeck A. "The Reciprocal Relationship Between Gratitude and Life Satisfaction: Evidence From Two Longitudinal Field Studies." *Frontiers in Psychology.* (2019 Nov 8);10:2480.
9. Patel A, Sharma PSVN, Kumar P. "Application of Mindfulness-Based Psychological Interventions in Infertility." *Journal of Human Reproductive Sciences.* (2020 Jan-Mar);13(1):3-21.
10. Smyth JM, Johnson JA, Auer BJ, Lehman E, Talamo G, Sciamanna CN. "Online Positive Affect Journaling in the Improvement of Mental Distress and Well-Being in General Medical Patients With Elevated Anxiety

Symptoms: A Preliminary Randomized Controlled Trial." *JMIR Mental Health.* (2018 Dec 10);5(4):e11290.

Acknowledgments

I am extremely grateful for the opportunity to write this book and to share my clinical experience with readers. This book would not have been possible without the support, guidance, and encouragement of countless people.

First and foremost, I would like to thank my patients who have allowed me to be a part of their fertility journey. Your trust, dedication, and resilience have been inspiring, and it has been an honor to work with you. Your feedback, questions, and concerns have helped me to understand the challenges you face and to develop strategies to overcome them.

I would also like to express my sincere gratitude to my enormous blended family, especially the children. I pray that I have been a good role model to you and that you know you can do anything, including blazing your own unconventional path. I promise you that you will not regret choosing a big, juicy life full of authenticity, good deeds, and inspiration. Go be great!

To my friends near and far, thank you all for loving and supporting me. You have given me, in equal measure, countless laughs and provocations for deep personal introspection. Both are important.

I could not do the work I do without the support and referrals from the obstetrics/gynecology and reproductive endocrinology communities in Los Angeles, CA. You have treated me like one of your own and I will always take excellent care of your patients. From the bottom of my heart, thank you.

I would like to thank the many experts in the field of acupuncture, fertility, and reproductive health for all of the good work that you do. Your documented findings made this book possible and have given me solid data with which I make my treatment plans.

And lastly, thank you to my Communications professors at DePaul University. You taught me the invaluable skills of critical thinking, clear expression, empathy, and powerful conveyance. I'll keep writing.

Thank you all.

Dr. Tamara ZumMallen, DAOM, L.Ac.
Beverly Hills, CA
May 19, 2023

Thank You For Reading *The Fertility Book*!
I really appreciate all of your feedback and
I love hearing what you have to say.

I would like your input to make the next version of this book and my future books better.

Please take two minutes now to leave a helpful review on Amazon letting me know what you thought of the book:
www.thefertilitybook.com/review

Thank you so very much!

Dr. Tamara ZumMallen, DAOM, L.Ac.

Made in the USA
Las Vegas, NV
04 January 2024